BIRTH

Introduction by Dr. Richard Hausknecht,
Associate Clinical Professor of Obstetrics and Gynecology,
Mount Sinai School of Medicine, New York

THOMAS Y. CROWELL COMPANY · ESTABLISHED 1834 · NEW YORK

BIRTH

PHOTOGRAPHS BY UWE AHRENS · TEXT BY JUDY CHOCK, CNM, AND
MARGARET MINER

Designed by Lynn Braswell

Manufactured in the United States of America

Library of Congress Cataloging in Publication Data

Ahrens, Uwe.
Birth.

Bibliography: p.
Includes index.
1. Childbirth. 2. Obstetrics—Popular works.
I. Chock, Judy, joint author. II. Miner, Margaret, joint author. III. Title.
RG525.A38   618'.4   77-2603
ISBN 0-690-01434-1 (H)

1 2 3 4 5 6 7 8 9 10

Contents

Acknowledgements

The pictures and captions in this book could not have come about without the generous cooperation of: Professor Dr. Gerhard Döring, head physician of the gynecological division of the Municipal Hospital of Munich-Harlaching; Dr. Knut Hanken, former head physician of the gynecological-obstetrical division of the Municipal Hospital of Munich-Harlaching; Dr. Jan-Diether Murken, head physician of the Children's Polyclinic of the University of Munich; Professor Dr. Klaus Riegel, head physician of the premature birth ward of the Children's Clinic of the University of Munich; Dr. Wolff von Weidenbach, head physician of the Private Gynecological Clinic of Munich; and Dr. Hans K. Wendl, head physician of the gynecological division of the District Hospital of Wedel, Hamburg.

We would also like to thank: doctors of the Rechts der Isar Gynecological Clinic at the Technical University of Munich; countless midwives and nurses; and above all the many marvelously human mothers, to whose openness these pictures bear witness.

And last but not least: Originally, nearly all of the photographs in this book were done on assignment for and published in the magazine *Eltern*, Munich. The material for the choice of pictures is mainly due to that assignment.

U. A. and K. R.

During the time I was preparing this manuscript many people offered their support and encouragement. I would like to thank first of all my clients for helping me understand more about the process of pregnancy and birth by sharing their first-hand experiences, for without their guidance my understanding of the birth cycle would be incomplete.

In the chapter on premature infants, Ramon J. C. Murphy, M.D., was of invaluable assistance in identifying and helping clarify for the scope of this book the pertinent information on the care of the high-risk newborn.

Finally, I would like to acknowledge Richard Hausknecht, M.D., my friend and associate, who freely offered his obstetrical expertise and reviewed the text.

J.L.C.

New York
August 1977

Introduction

Couples in recent years have shown a marked desire to increase their understanding and awareness of conception, pregnancy, and birth. This book combines a series of excellent photographs with a well-written text that begins with a clear and simple discussion of conception and carefully reviews the various stages of a normal pregnancy. The many major and minor physiological changes that regularly occur are explained—a sure method of relieving the anxieties that plague every couple about to have a child.

It has always been difficult to explain with words alone the actual process of a normal birth. Most of the available films, including those shown on television, are only suggestive of reality. The photographs in this book, a superb graphic teaching instrument in themselves, combined with the text, give a total picture of the childbirth process from conception to birth.

The text addresses itself to this desire on the part of young couples to both experience and understand childbirth, exploring the roles of husband, wife, labor monitrice, and doctor during the various stages of the process. In addition, different theories of childbirth are discussed, such as Grantly Dick-Read's theory of "prepared childbirth," Lamaze's "psychoprophylaxis," as well as the more recent ideas of Leboyer. There is no question that these obstetricians and the methods they have proposed have had a significant impact on modern obstetrics; one result is that the use of heavy sedation and anesthesia has been reduced significantly so couples are now able to share the excitement of childbirth together as well as those moving first moments with their newborn child.

While pictures and explanations are what this book is all about, hearing the actual words of the patients who have "already been there" is particularly reassuring and comforting. It is calming to know that others have shared similar fears and joys.

Modern American obstetrics is changing fairly rapidly, fetal monitoring is becoming a nationwide standard, anesthetic techniques have been improved, many couples are requesting formal childbirth classes which have markedly reduced the necessity for routine anesthesia during delivery, and midwives are once again assuming an important role in the care of the pregnant woman. The advent of antepartum fetal monitoring techniques, amniotic fluid studies, and sonography has made it possible for diabetic women, Rh-sensitized women, hypertensive women, and older women to bear healthy children.

The more solid information that each couple has about pregnancy, labor, and delivery, the better able will they be to make important decisions about the choice of a doctor, midwife, childbirth classes, medication, and place of delivery. This important book provides much of the basic information necessary to make the experience of having a child exciting, unique, and healthy.

DR. RICHARD HAUSKNECHT
Associate Clinical Professor of Obstetrics and Gynecology,
Mount Sinai School of Medicine, New York

Pregnancy

Each pregnancy is different. Each woman's experience is unique. No one else can tell you exactly what you will feel. Your body, though, will guide you well. Pregnancy is a time to pay attention to your body's needs.

Some women feel marvelous almost throughout pregnancy. Others feel miserable. Twenty years ago women were constantly told to rest and be careful, which was frustrating for the woman who wanted to be out playing tennis. Today, many women think they're supposed to be active into the ninth month, working and keeping a beautiful home as well. This is fairly difficult if you feel a desperate need for twelve hours' sleep a day. If you do feel ill and tired, take all the rest you want. And report the fatigue to your doctor. But don't worry that it's a bad sign. Every day marvelously healthy babies are born to women who felt awful as well as to ones who felt terrific during pregnancy.

Pregnancy begins with conception, of course. Unfortunately there's no convenient way of telling when conception has taken place. So a woman who's trying to become pregnant should avoid medicines (even be cautious in the use of aspirin and antacids). You may be several weeks pregnant before you're aware of it, and the first eight weeks of development are particularly crucial. For this reason it's best not to expose the fetus to any medication.

Conception may take place whenever a woman is fertile, which is usually about midway between menstrual cycles, at the time of ovulation. Ovulation occurs when stimulation of the ovaries by pituitary hormones results in the rupture of a ripe ovum, or egg cell, from one ovary. The ovum has a life of about twelve to twenty-four hours.

A common symptom of ovulation is lower abdominal pain on one side or the other (depending on which ovary is involved). This discomfort is called "Mittelschmerz," and if you experience it, you know when you ovulate. A more precise method is to keep a record of your basal body temperature. Drugstores carry special basal ther-

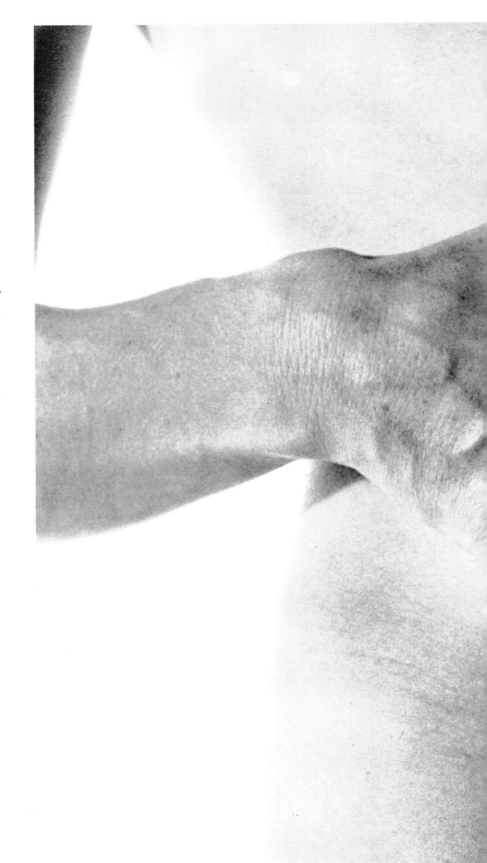

When a woman feels a new life within her, her thoughts and feelings revolve around the baby and herself. She is evolving a new identity.

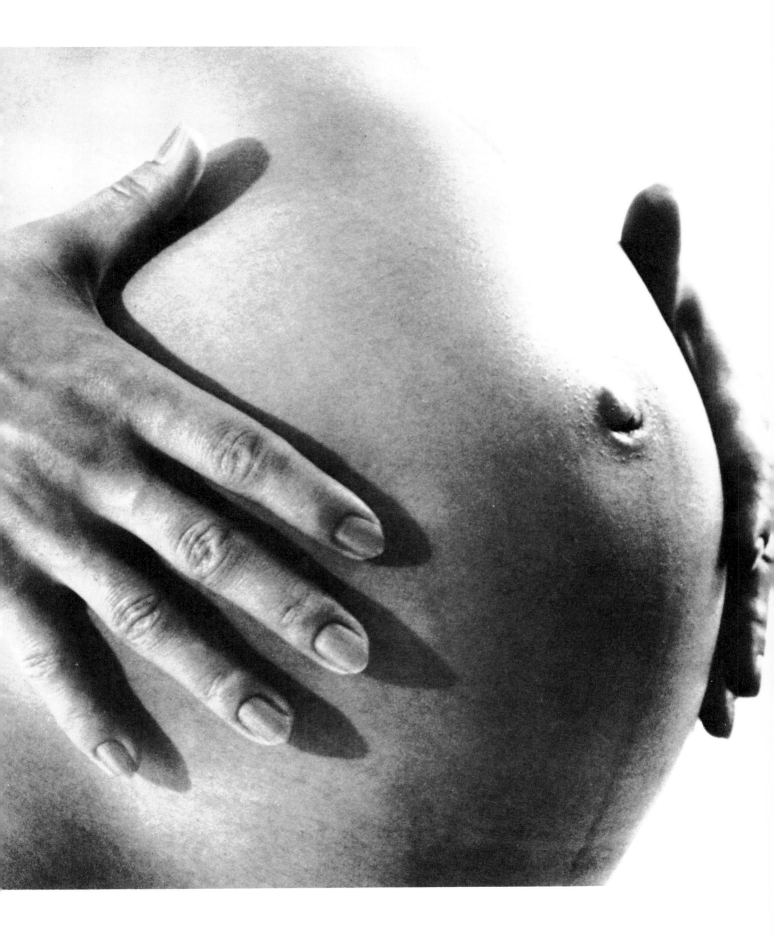

mometers that come with instructions and a chart. You take your temperature at the same time every morning, before getting up or talking. A shift upward in temperature will occur following ovulation. Typically, in the preovulation phase, the morning temperature will be rather low, about a degree below normal. When ovulation occurs, your temperature will rise about a degree. If you have sexual intercourse around this time, fertilization of the ovum may take place. If it does not, then your menstrual period will begin in approximately fourteen days. With a temperature chart you will have some indication very quickly of whether you're pregnant. If your temperature remains at the high level associated with ovulation, you're probably pregnant. If it drops back to the lower level, you're probably not.

If you have a temperature chart, keep it. It can be useful toward the end of pregnancy if there's a question about when the baby's due.

The normal male ejaculate of 1½ to 3 millimeters of seminal fluid contains 60 million or more sperm per millimeter, each with a life of approximately twenty-four to thirty-six hours. It is necessary for only one of these sperm to unite with the ovum for fertilization to take place. Nevertheless, a normally fertile couple may try for six months or a year or perhaps even longer before conceiving. The ideal frequency of intercourse for conception is about every other day. (More frequent ejaculation may lower the sperm count.) If you've been having intercourse fairly frequently at the times you're fertile, and haven't conceived in the course of a year, consider consulting a doctor skilled in treating fertility problems.

The joining of sperm and ovum usually takes place in the Fallopian tube leading from the ovary to the uterus. The resulting embryo is moved by wavelike movements of the tube, and reaches the uterus in about seven days. From the time of fertilization until about six to eight weeks later, when the placenta is fully developed, the embryo's life is maintained by estrogens and progesterone produced by the corpus luteum; this is a specialized mass of tissue that forms in the ovary at the site from which the egg ruptured.

The average duration of pregnancy, counting from the first day of the last menstrual period, is about 280 days, or 40 weeks. The first apparent sign of pregnancy is usually a missed or scanty menstrual period. You can calculate your estimated date of confinement (often abbreviated EDC) by counting back three months from the first day of your last period and adding seven days. For example, if your last period began on September 10, the EDC would be June 17. The calculation can be simplified by designating the months by numbers. Then, the foregoing example becomes 9/10 minus three months equals 6/10 plus seven days is 6/17. The estimate is only approximate, but about forty percent of women go into labor within five days of the EDC, and nearly two-thirds do so within ten days.

Other presumptive signs of pregnancy include enlargement and tenderness in the breasts; a change in the color of the mucuous membranes of the vagina and vulva from pink to a bluish purple, and increased pigmentation of the skin, most noticeably in a line extending from the navel to the pubic hair and around the nipples.

If your period is more than three weeks late and you might be pregnant, this is the time to make an appointment with an obstetrician or at an obstetrical clinic to be sure your diagnosis is correct and to discuss the probable course of the pregnancy, and whether any problems might be anticipated. A urine or blood test for pregnancy can be done, and a positive result is a very probable sign of pregnancy. Also a physician or nurse-midwife can detect by pelvic examination an enlargement and softening of the uterus and a slight darkening of the color of the cervix, both of which indicate a probable pregnancy. Technically, there are only three signs that are positive proof of pregnancy: detection of the fetal heartbeat; perception of active fetal movement by a trained examiner; recognition of the fetus, by X-ray or sonographic examination.

THE FIRST TRIMESTER

Pregnancy is frequently described in terms of trimesters. The first trimester is the first thirteen weeks of development; the second extends from fourteen to twenty-seven weeks; and the third from twenty-eight weeks to forty weeks. at which time the baby is said to have reached term.

Fetal growth takes place at an extraordinarily rapid rate. An adult weighs about twenty-three times what he did at birth, but a newborn infant weighs about six billion times what he did at conception. Within this period he has changed structurally from a single-celled organism to a complex of organ systems which can support life outside the mother's body.

By four weeks of gestation, the foundations of all the organs have been laid, including the heart and digestive system. But the embryo is still only $3/16$ of an inch long.

At six weeks, the placenta has begun to develop, and the embryo is now floating in a small, fluid-filled sac formed by two membranes, the amnion and the chorion. The amniotic fluid, which is produced from the placenta and the embryo, protects the new life from jars and jolts. It's such an excellent insulator that it's rare for even a severe fall by the mother to harm the developing baby.

Ordinarily the amniotic sac remains intact until sometime after labor begins, but occasionally it will rupture earlier (this may happen in any trimester). Your doctor's treatment would depend partially on the age of the fetus at the time, the main concern being to avoid premature delivery or infection. Occasionally the sac heals spontaneously, and no treatment at all is required. If the rupture takes place at term, most often labor contractions begin within twenty-four hours.

By the seventh week of gestation, the fetus has developed tiny buds for arms and legs. The umbilical cord is lengthening (it will be about eighteen to twenty inches at term). The placenta is beginning to perform the work of providing nourishment to the fetus and removing waste products.

The developing placenta is vital to the well-being of the baby. It is the organ that mediates between mother and fetus, being attached to the mother's uterine wall and to the fetus via the umbilical cord. In the placenta there is an exchange of substances between the blood vessels of the mother and those of the baby. The very fine cellular structure of the placenta allows only some of the components of the mother's blood to be passed to the baby as nourishment. All the fetal wastes are carried through the umbilical cord to the placenta where they are picked up by the mother's circulatory system and excreted by her lungs and kidneys.

It is the placenta that produces the hormone (chorionic gonadotropin) that is looked for in pregnancy tests. While the placenta is still developing, this hormone stimulates the corpus luteum to produce estrogens and progesterone. After six weeks of pregnancy, however, the placenta is able to take over the work of the corpus luteum (which starts regressing) and the production of chorionic gonadotropin is somewhat reduced.

The placenta is expelled following the birth of the baby as the "afterbirth."

Eight weeks is considered the end of the embryonic period and the beginning of the fetal period. The fetus is now about 1⅛ inches long. Virtually all the major structures of the body have taken their basic form. Subsequent development consists primarily in the growth and maturation of the already differentiated cells representing the various organs.

What does the mother experience during this first trimester? If she has been looking forward to having a child, she is usually elated to find she is pregnant. But even the proudest mothers may have some bad days; for many women find this trimester the most difficult period of a pregnancy. There are inevitable worries over whether the pregnancy will go well, and often worries over the changes it will bring in the parents' lives. And there may be some physical discomfort—early pregnancy may feel like a continuation and intensification of premenstrual malaise, and it is in the first two months that the mother is most apt to experience morning sickness, which despite its name can occur in the afternoon and evening, too.

The cause of morning sickness isn't known. One theory is that it's simply the result of the very rapid growth of the embryo and uterus. However, if you have it, there are two consolations. One, it's somewhat functional. You may find that you can't stand cigarette smoke, alcohol or staying up late. A healthy life is forced upon you. Second, morning sickness doesn't last forever. You *will* feel better soon. In the meantime, a traditional cure for the nausea is a piece of cracker or dry toast and a rest. And, generally, a light carbohydrate diet is recommended for breakfast (cereal and toast, not bacon and eggs).

Frequent vomiting should be reported to your doctor, for it can cause imbalances in the body's metabolism. Treatment includes fluid replacement, diet control and rest. However, such a problem is rare.

Although you won't begin to "show" in the first trimester, you will start gaining weight and your uterus will be growing. Estrogens (produced by the ovaries, placenta and adrenal glands) cause a thickening of the uterine musculature, a similar development of the endometrium (the lining of the uterus) and an increase in the pelvic blood supply. The original size of the uterus is 3 to 4 inches in length and 1½ to 2 inches in width at the fundus (the top). By the end of this trimester it will be about the size of a medium grapefruit. You'll probably become aware of its growth by a common symptom: frequent urination and perhaps an occasional slight loss of control. This is caused by pressure of the uterus on the bladder. It will ease later.

The estrogens also stimulate breast development, with the breasts becoming larger and more tender as the milk ducts develop and the aureoles around the nipples becoming larger and darker (they will return to their original color appearance after pregnancy). Wearing a good bra will help the breasts retain their resiliency.

Progesterone (produced in the ovaries, placenta and adrenal glands) also stimulates the growth of the uterus; and it inhibits contraction of smooth muscles, especially in the uterus but throughout the body as well. Thus progesterone plays a role in guarding against contractions of the uterus that might lead to premature labor, but it affects the smooth muscles of the digestive tract as well, leading to sluggish digestion and constipation. If you're taking iron (and it's prescribed for most pregnant women), this aggravates the constipation. You can control this constipation by taking extra fluids, especially juices like prune juice, and a tablespoon of bran in the evening. Don't use a laxative without consulting your doctor.

The relaxation of the pyloric sphincter muscle between the stomach and the duodenum (the beginning of the small intestine) can result in an occasional backward flow of food into the stomach, which means heartburn. Along about the seventh month of pregnancy, a big chili dinner can be a big mistake, for some women. You can ease the pain by eating small amounts of food frequently and avoiding spicy or acid foods. If necessary, use a nonsodium antacid (your doctor will recommend one). Don't use bicarbonate of soda or any of the bubbling antacids, because of their high sodium content.

Early in pregnancy there are many important changes in the production of ovarian and adrenal hormones. One of the changes associated with the increased production of estrogens and cortisol is increased insulin utilization. This may give rise to an elevated blood sugar which can contribute to the development of a mild diabetes in some pregnant women. If you or anyone in your family has ever had diabetes or a similar condition, you should have a glucose-tolerance test in the first trimester.

Finally, although the jokes about the strange appetites of pregnant women are exaggerated and boring, you *will* feel hungry. If your diet is balanced, you probably can eat all you want with only healthy results. For those who enjoy food, this is one of the pleasures of pregnancy.

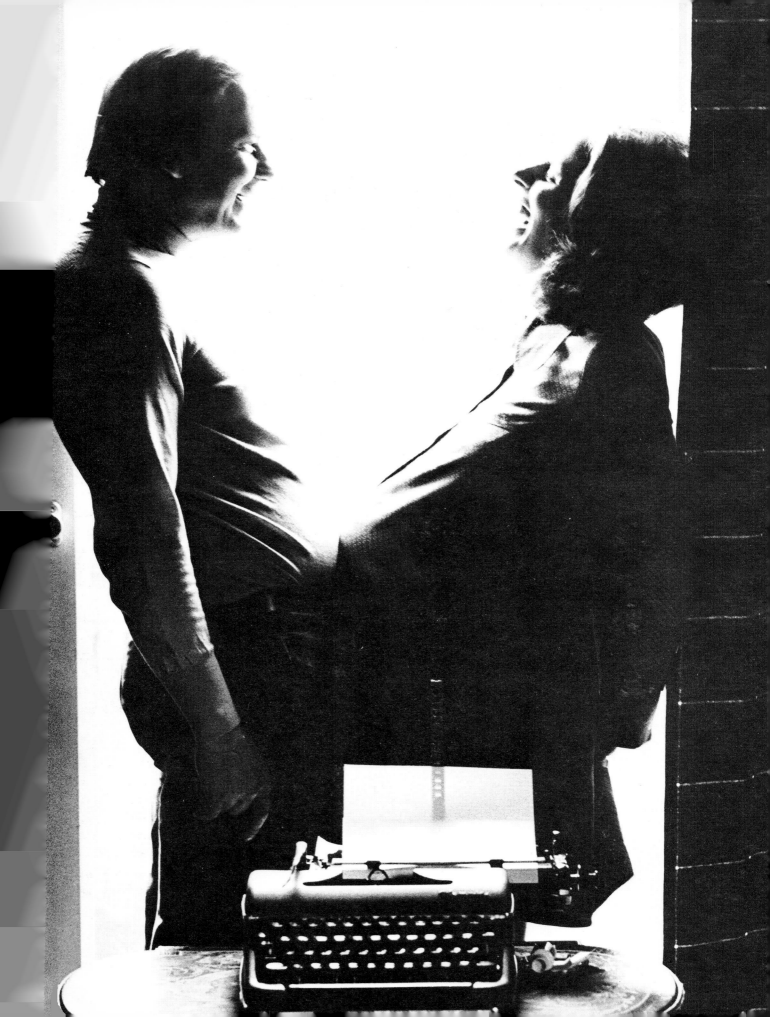

THE SECOND TRIMESTER

In these months, the fetus will grow from a length of about three inches and a weight of about one ounce to eleven to fourteen inches in length and over a pound in weight. In the third month of gestation, the fingers and toes are differentiated and the nails begin to form. The external genitalia begin to show characteristics of male or female sex. In the fourth month, by using special instruments, the heartbeat can usually be picked up. The fetal head is disproportionately large, but the eyes, ears, nose and mouth are approaching their typical appearance. In the fifth month, the fetus's transparent skin is covered with lanugo (a fine hair) and some scalp hair is evident. In the sixth month, the skin has become wrinkled and is covered with vernix (a creamy coating). Fat is first being deposited beneath the skin. The eyelids have separated and the eyelashes have formed.

For the mother, the second trimester may be a very good time. Many women feel especially energetic and well in this period. It is at this time, somewhere around eighteen weeks, that fetal movement is first felt by the mother. The first sensations may be very faint, like a slight scratching or rumble of the stomach. They soon become stronger, and some babies are so active that by seven months they seem to be trying to kick their way out.

Once the fetus is fully active, if you feel her moving a couple of times a day or more, this is a good sign. However, it's extremely easy to miss normal movement if you're busy and distracted, even by a routine activity such as shopping. You may all of a sudden have a scary feeling that the fetus hasn't stirred in several days, when in fact she has been moving as usual. Therefore, most doctors are not concerned if a woman reports anxiety over lack of movement, particularly early in pregnancy. Their normal response is to suggest that fetal activity will be felt again in a day, and this is usually what happens.

In the fifth month, the uterus starts to rise into the abdominal cavity, relieving some of the pressure on the bladder and the need for frequent urination.

In this trimester, you may feel a periodic sharp pain in the lower abdomen, usually on one side only. (This pain is extremely variable and may occur at any time in pregnancy.) It's nothing to worry about. The rapid growth of the fetus and uterus puts tension on the round ligaments on each side of the uterus that attach it to the pubic bone; as a result, these ligaments sometimes go into a brief spasm.

Toward the middle or end of the third trimester, it will probably become apparent that you're pregnant, not just gaining weight. This spares you appraising looks and the need for explanation. However, T-shirts labeled "baby" are popular in the transition period.

Up until fairly recently, women were often urged not to gain more than twenty pounds at most during pregnancy. This left a lot of women hungry. Actually, a gain of twenty to twenty-five pounds seems to be normal and desirable. But because overweight is associated with a condition called preeclampsia, or toxemia, it was formerly hoped that dieting would help prevent this condition from developing.

In general, in the second and third trimesters a pregnant woman needs an additional 200 calories a day, assuming her level of activity remains the same. By the end of pregnancy a weight gain of nearly 18 pounds can be accounted for on the basis of physiological changes: growth of the fetus (7½ pounds), uterus (2 pounds) and the placenta (1 pound); production of amniotic fluid (2 pounds); an increase in blood (3½ pounds); breast and milk development (1½ pounds). An additional gain of 2 to 3 pounds results from the retention of fluids in the pelvis and legs; this edema is due to decreased circulation caused by the pressure of the uterus.

Toward the end of the second trimester, you may feel some difficulty in breathing or a slight malaise in the region of the heart or even heart palpitations. These sensations are all normal. They're caused by an increase in the respiratory rate needed to excrete the extra carbon dioxide produced by the fetus; by an increase of about forty percent in the blood volume; and by upward pressure by the uterus.

Because of the relaxing effect of progesterone, there is a loss of tone in the bladder and ureters, which predisposes the urinary system toward infection. To counteract this, drink plenty of fluids (cranberry juice is very good for maintaining proper acidity) and urinate whenever you feel any urge. Holding back causes overdistention of the bladder, and it becomes more difficult to empty it completely.

THE THIRD TRIMESTER

The fetus is rapidly gaining the weight and size it will need to survive in the outside world. In the seventh month, while the organs are continuing to develop, the baby's weight will double and he will grow about three inches longer. At the end of the eighth month, the baby will weigh 4½ to 5½ pounds and be 16 to 18 inches long. (There's an old fallacy that an eight-month baby has a lesser chance of surviving a premature birth than a seven-month baby. On the contrary, the older baby's chances are much better.) In the ninth month, the baby becomes more rotund, thanks to the deposit of fat under the skin; this fat is going to be needed for insulation. The final maturation of all the organs, especially the nervous system, is taking place.

At term, the average baby girl weighs 7 pounds and the average boy weighs 7½. The skin of the body is smooth and occasionally has some lanugo (fine hair) on the shoulders and back. The scalp is covered with dark hairs. The fingers and toes have well-developed nails, which project beyond their tips. The bones of the head are well ossified, although the "soft spot" will remain for another twelve to eighteen months. The eyes are usually a uniform slate color, which often will change later. Black babies have a dusky, bluish-red color of skin at birth, which may not at all suggest the darker pigmentation they may assume in a few weeks. White babies appear very pale, and may have blue-tinged hands and feet before a more pink tone develops.

For the mother, the third trimester may seem a very long time. The woman who hasn't given birth before is especially likely to be affected by a mood of anticipation with apprehension. It's like waiting for Christmas. Time moves slowly.

The baby is now always a presence, so large and often so active that you can't forget him or her for long. The sensation of having another being inside you can be disorienting as well as exciting. Your body that was previously all you is now part someone else. You look in the mirror, and you don't look like yourself.

At some point in these last months, almost all women begin to long to be thin again and able to move freely. The physically active woman may particularly resent being slow and heavy. As much as you may be enjoying the pregnancy, the sheer physical burden may become oppressive at some point. Try to make all preparations for the arrival of the baby early in this trimester, and get other work cleared up so you can forget about it later if necessary. Some women sail up and into labor without a break in their normal activity. For others there comes a day when they just want to stay in bed or go to the movies. Indulge yourself. The woman who approaches birth rested and fresh is much more likely to enjoy the experience.

In the third trimester, many women find it hard to get a good night's sleep because of the weight of the uterus and the movement of the baby. Keep a good book or crossword puzzle by your bed, and make up for lost sleep with a nap if necessary. Don't worry that sleeping on your stomach will hurt the baby. It won't. However, it may become impossible. A side position is usually easiest, perhaps with a pillow to support the abdomen.

Edema, or swelling, of the feet and legs, is very common, and should be treated by resting with your legs raised. If it's severe enough to interfere with normal walking or causes any significant pain, wear supporting elastic stockings.

Varicose veins may become prominent at any time in pregnancy, but especially now. Prolonged standing will aggravate the condition. Again, the treatment is primarily rest with raised legs and the use of elastic stockings. Varicosities of the vulva are relieved by wearing a sanitary pad held by an elastic belt. Hemorrhoids are also aggravated by pregnancy. The pain and swelling can usually be reduced by use of a topical anesthetic and a stool softener, which your doctor will recommend, and by warm soaks.

At some point in the third trimester, usually in the eighth month, you'll begin to experience false labor (Braxton-Hicks) contractions, which are randomly timed, virtually painless uterine contractions. They are a rather strange sensation at first, and when they get stronger, they may be confused with the start of labor. They are, however, only toning-up exercises (true labor is described at the beginning of the next chapter).

The unglamorous discomforts of the third trimester may take the romance out of pregnancy. A sense of fun helps. If you haven't laughed much lately, make a point of having some dinners out, going to the movies, seeing friends.

At term, or in the last two weeks of pregnancy, the uterus descends, and projects lower and farther forward. This brings relative ease in breathing and comfort after eating. The head or presenting part of the baby descends in the pelvis, increasing the stress on the cervix, which may begin to show the flattening out, or effacement, that precedes birth. Braxton-Hicks contractions are more frequent. You are ready to have your baby.

Prospective parents are naturally concerned about general health in pregnancy, and the first thing to remember is that pregnancy itself is a healthy state. Many women feel their best during pregnancy. The physical stress may bring on some of the discomforts we've mentioned, but these are usually no more significant than stiff muscles would be after a lot of physical exercise.

Today, there's very little emphasis on restricting activity in pregnancy. It's no longer believed that skiing or swimming or other popular kinds of exercise are at all dangerous early in pregnancy. Somewhere in the second trimester, your body (and probably your doctor) will let you know you should slow down.

Don't force yourself to keep going when you're very tired. In pregnancy your stamina may change suddenly, so that one day you're full of energy and the next you want two naps. Try to get all the sleep you want. If you develop a cold, flu, cystitis or any fever, report it to your doctor and take extra good care of yourself. But, again, don't take cold tablets or other medication on your own. Ask your doctor's advice.

Be especially aware of how you move. Don't bend from the waist when lifting packages or young children. Squat down and then raise the weight, using your leg muscles instead of your back muscles. Don't stand leaning backward to compensate for the weight of your abdomen. This, too, strains the back muscles. Instead, keep your spine straight and let the uterus drop forward. If you have a history of back strain, mention this to your doctor. He may suggest an exercise, such as the fifth body-building exercise listed in our chapter on prepared birth. Simple leg lifts will strengthen your abdominal and leg muscles. Don't do "sitting-up" exercises, which may cause a separation of the muscles along the midline of the abdomen.

There's no reason to limit sexual intercourse at any time during a normal pregnancy. A woman's sexual desires may vary and fluctuate in pregnancy (partly for physiological reasons) and the man's sexual interests may be influenced by concern about his new role as a father and all the various adjustments he has to make. It's also common for the man to worry about injuring the fetus, especially once he's become aware of its movement; however, such an injury is virtually impossible. Try to be open with each other about any problems, and try not to become too anxious about mood changes that may pass very quickly. Ask your doctor about anything that concerns you. A harmonious sexual relationship between the parents is a benefit to the child, too.

Couples often ask whether any particular sexual position is medically preferable. There is none, but toward the end of pregnancy the male superior position may become uncomfortable or impossible. As to whether intercourse might cause a spontaneous abortion, it was thought in the recent past that prostaglandins in the man's seminal fluid might stimulate uterine contractions. But there is no evidence to back up this theory. Today, a pregnant woman is asked to avoid intercouse only when there is vaginal bleeding or some other indication that a spontaneous abortion might occur and at the end of pregnancy when the cervix has started to dilate. The only warnings are to be very careful not to get any bacteria from the region of the anus into the area of the vagina. And air should *never* be blown into the vagina; it can enter the woman's bloodstream via the placenta, an occurrence which is extremely dangerous.

Washing the genitals frequently with mild soap and water is the best method of keeping them clean and free of bacteria. Because there is a greater discharge of mucus in pregnancy, cotton underpants are more comfortable than synthetic materials. Silk and synthetics are nice but tend to aggravate vaginitis—at all times, not just in pregnancy.

Douching is never normally needed at any time and is completely contraindicated in pregnancy. Damage can be done by the water pressure or the hard tip. Far from protecting against infection, it may introduce it.

Your druggist may try to sell you special ointments for the breasts and abdomen that are supposed to prevent striae, or stretch marks. There's no proof these do any good. Regular use of a standard lotion or moisturizer is as effective as anything else. A well-fitted bra supporting the breasts is a help. Occasionally a pelvic girdle is prescribed to support the abdomen and back.

A sonographic examination. As the technician moves the scope, the picture shows up on the screen to the left. The machine will also print a sonogram, as shown below.

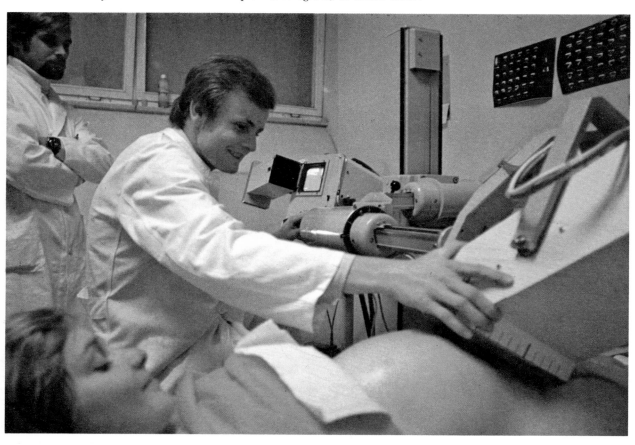

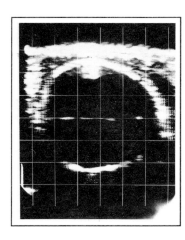

A section of a sonogram, show-ing the abdominal wall and fetal head.

You should wash your breasts, especially the nipples and aureoles, with mild soap and water to prevent the crusting of colostrum (the thin yellow liquid that forms prior to milk). If you plan to breast feed, it's advisable to massage the breasts daily in the last two months to express the colostrum so it won't block the milk ducts. Squeeze the breasts behind the areola in a pumping fashion. Rubbing the nipples with a towel will harden them in preparation for nursing. However, if you're lazy about all this and want to breast feed, go ahead with it. You'll undoubtedly be successful.

Bathing and showering is fine at any time, even at term after the cervix has started to dilate. As long as the amniotic membrane is intact, it's impossible for bath water to come in contact with the fetus. The real danger in bathing is falling and hurting yourself. Late in pregnancy it's easy to lose your balance. Be very careful.

Today, health standards in pregnancy emphasize restricting exposure to medicines, X-rays, nicotine and other drugs. German measles, which is dangerous in the first three months of pregnancy, is much less of a problem now that a vaccine is available. Toxoplasmosis, another otherwise mild disease that may be dangerous to the fetus, is best avoided by not handling cat litter or feces and by not eating rare or raw meat.

It was only at the time of the thalidomide tragedy in 1961–62 that doctors began to realize the serious effect medicines may have in pregnancy. As already emphasized, all medicines should be avoided if possible. Cigarette smoking should be cut back, preferably cut out. The babies of smokers are smaller at term. Alcohol also passes through the placenta and can affect the fetus. Heavy drinking isn't advisable, especially on a daily basis. Marijuana hasn't been associated with any particular problems, but it hasn't been carefully studied. A good general rule is to avoid substance use of any kind.

Dental work can safely be done in pregnancy but X-rays should be postponed. Novocaine or the like is fine but not nitrous oxide (laughing gas). There's no truth to the notion that having a baby causes cavities. In the last twelve weeks of pregnancy the fetus does require substantial amounts of calcium as his skeleton develops, but calcium is drawn from the mother's bones, not teeth.

In the last trimester, your doctor may recommend X-rays to determine whether your pelvic passage is wide enough for the baby's head. In such a case, the benefit of the knowledge far outweighs the almost negligible risk. But, in general, X-rays should not be done in pregnancy, especially early in pregnancy.

Most doctors prescribe vitamins and minerals in pregnancy, particularly folic acid and iron. This is a good precaution, for nutritional imbalances are more apt to occur during pregnancy. Vitamins and minerals should be taken with a juice that contains vitamin C (such as orange, grapefruit or tomato juice); this promotes their absorption. Eat a well-balanced diet with milk or a milk product each day. A good prenatal diet is associated with healthier, stronger mothers and babies.

Selecting the most appropriate type of medical care for yourself and your baby is very important. Alternatives include care by a single doctor or group of doctors; care in a hospital-based clinic, which can be very good in some hospitals; and care through a prepaid health plan. Excellent care can also be obtained through a Certified Nurse-Midwife (CNM) and physician team. The CNMs are now on the staffs of many large teaching hospitals and also in joint practice with private doctors. If you're interested in prepared childbirth, there's a chapter on this ahead.

If you don't already have an obstetrician you like, a good place to start is by talking to couples who've recently had children. Try to find out what kind of rapport they were able to establish with their doctors or midwives during pregnancy and what their experiences were during labor and delivery.

Call up the medical people you're interested in. How the office staff responds is often a clue to the attitudes of the medical staff. Do the people you talk to answer your questions easily? Do they call back when they say they will? Don't hesitate to ask about fees. Does the fee include classes in prepared childbirth or attendance of a coach during the labor and delivery if you want this? Will the fee be higher for a Caesarian or in any other special situation?

Prepared childbirth classes are usually extra, but a concerned doctor can tell you where he refers patients and what the cost will be. If he can't do this immediately, be warned that he may not be interested in this method.

Hospital fees vary, especially in large cities, but a stay of two to four days may equal or exceed the cost of your doctor. Ask if the hospital has modern fetal monitoring equipment and an intensive care unit for newborns (small, local hospitals may not have such units, but they should have clear procedures for the transfer of babies when necessary). Also find out what kind of anesthesia service is available and if it is available at all hours.

Speak with your doctor. The more you do, the more you can learn about him or her and the more the doctor can learn about you and how to help you have the kind of experience you want. If you can't establish a comfortable relationship, consider trying another doctor. You don't need a doctor who's a buddy, but you do need one with whom you can work.

On your first visit, your doctor should record your complete general history, with the object of identifying any condition that might affect your present pregnancy. He will probably ask you about your family background; your physical and emotional well-being; past medical and surgical history; your menstrual history, including when you started menstruating, how often you menstruate and for how many days; and a complete account of any past gynecological and obstetrical problems. Finally, he will record information on this pregnancy and the date of your last menstrual period.

Your physical exam should include weight, blood pressure and a urine test for the presence of protein and sugar. Protein may indicate a problem with kidney function, sugar with glucose metabolism. In addition to a general check of your heart, lungs and so on, you will be given a pelvic exam to determine the size of your uterus and pelvic structure. If you've never had a vaginal examination before, tell this to your doctor. He or she should be gentle and explain the procedure. If something really bothers you, say so. If you definitely don't like the way your doctor talks or acts at this time, maybe you should change to another doctor.

Your doctor will probably take a Pap smear and do a blood test for type and Rh factor, for hemoglobin and hematocrit, for syphilis (required by law in most states), and a rubella titre. A glucose-tolerance test should be scheduled if your history includes any of the following: previous diabetes in pregnancy; obesity; diabetes in your family; recurrent sugar in your urine; if you've had a previous infant weighing nine pounds or more, or if you've given birth to a stillborn infant or one with a serious defect.

This test involves drinking a glass of fluid rich in glucose and then having blood taken every hour for several hours. You may feel woozy and you'll certainly be bored. It's best to have someone along with you if possible. The test, though, is very important, and can alert the doctor to problems that may arise later. Diabetics and their babies tend to have special difficulties, and if you do have a problem with sugar metabolism you should have your baby in a hospital with a good perinatal service. With up-to-date care the chances of avoiding any serious complications are excellent.

Your doctor will probably ask you to come in once a month for about seven months and then every two weeks, and then every week in the ninth month. At each visit he'll check your blood pressure, urine, weight, growth of the uterus, any swelling of your hands or legs and the fetal heartbeat. In the last month of pregnancy you may also be given a pelvic exam each visit to determine the baby's position and size and whether there are any changes in your cervix indicating the approach of the onset of labor.

The great majority of pregnancies proceed without complications through the birth of a healthy baby to a healthy mother. However, as every intelligent woman knows, problems can arise. And if they do, many women feel bitter that they weren't warned. Doctors and midwives are almost invariably reassuring and optimistic on the theory that it's wrong to provoke anxieties in the mother-to-be. However, most pregnant women are at least as capable as their doctors of adjusting to reality.

Medical people shouldn't feel embarrassed in discussing problems in pregnancy, for advances in obstetrical medicine have dramatically improved the chances of diagnosing and treating such problems. Most women now properly expect that pregnancy and birth will be rewarding experiences. In the past, childbearing was often properly dreaded. Mere survival was an achievement. We still have a long way to go, but we've also come a long way.

The most common of the serious problems is spontaneous abortion in the first trimester. This occurs in about ten to fifteen percent of pregnancies. In most cases the cause is a major error in early development—a chromosomal defect which is not preventable. In the past, many doctors treated such situations with various hormones in the mistaken belief that these pregnancies could be "saved." It has become apparent that such medications do no good whatsoever and may even damage a developing fetus. Most often there is no repetition of the difficulty in the next pregnancy, but if a woman has two or more spontaneous abortions in a row (especially if they follow a similar pattern), she should seek help from a clinic or doctor specializing in problematic pregnancies. The chances that she can be helped are good.

A spontaneous abortion, or miscarriage, is typically preceded by bleeding and often cramping. These symptoms should always be reported to your doctor. You may be advised to avoid sexual intercourse and physical exertion. However, in the first trimester, these restrictions are largely just precautions, and the woman who does abort shouldn't feel that it could have been prevented by more rest or chastity.

A small percentage of pregnancy loss is caused by ectopic, or tubal, pregnancy, in which the ovum becomes implanted in the Fallopian tube. At some point in the first twelve weeks, the tube will rupture unless there has been surgical intervention. The symptoms of ectopic pregnancy are severe abdominal pain on one side and light spotting. If the tube does rupture, surgery is required to control the bleeding.

Bleeding is not necessarily a sign of impending abortion. Spotting and even bleeding may simply pass. Bright red bleeding in any trimester may be caused by erosion of the cervix resulting from a simple vaginal infection, such as monilia or trichomonas. In the first trimester, bleeding may occur about the time of the first missed menstrual period; it's caused by the ovum embedding in the uterine lining. At about ten to twelve weeks gestation, there may be spotting as the corpus luteum recedes. All bleeding should be promptly reported to your doctor.

There is occasionally bleeding late in pregnancy, in most cases without pain and without any serious consequences. However, bleeding in the late second or third trimester may indicate placenta previa, a condition in which the placenta is located low in the uterus, partially or completely covering the cervical opening. As the cervix effaces (flattens out), the blood vessels of the placenta are exposed and there is bleeding into the vagina. The condition is dangerous because of the risk of sudden and severe hemorrhage from the placenta. Bed rest is required, and if possible the woman should not be left alone. At least she should always be in reach of a telephone, and arrangements should be made for quick transport to the hospital. Delivery is usually by Caesarian section.

In the third trimester, there is sometimes a pink-tinged discharge as the cervix softens and small blood vessels break. This is no cause for alarm. Birth is near.

Toxemia, or preeclampsia, is another serious condition. It's a disease process that occurs only in pregnancy and the cause is unknown. We know only that it's most apt to affect younger women who are having their first child and who are in a state of poor nutrition. The symptoms are swelling of the face and fingers (as well as legs and ankles), elevated blood pressure, severe or continuous headache, sometimes dimness or blurring of vision and protein in the urine. It may result in an underdeveloped placenta and a small, poorly nourished baby. Severe cases may cause the mother to have convulsions and lead to the death of the baby. Treatment is usually bed rest, an adequate diet and sedation to aid in obtaining rest. The aim is to decrease the stress on the mother and increase her circulation, specifically to the uterus, placenta and fetus.

Report to your doctor any strong, constant pain in your abdomen or chest. It may be caused by some innocent factor, such as the fetus kicking, or in the third trimester, harmless cramping low in the pelvis, over the pubic bone, as the cervix starts to efface. If you have noticed a swollen, warm, tender spot on your leg or in your groin, don't massage such a spot; it might dislodge a blood clot. The treatment for this is usually bed rest and anticoagulant therapy.

In diagnosing difficulties, sonography is an invaluable and frequently used technique, which is completely safe for mother and baby. A sonographic examination can be performed in ten minutes. Essentially it involves using sonic (sound) waves to get a "picture" of the uterus and fetus. You simply lie down on a couch or stretcher and a nurse or technician rubs your abdomen with mineral oil, which helps conduct the sonic waves. A technician then moves a device that looks like a small microphone across your abdomen. It transmits high-frequency sound waves, which are bounced back and transmitted to a machine that translates them into a picture that somewhat resembles an X-ray. The technician is trained to interpret this.

The picture usually shows the fetal head, the placenta, uterus, abdominal wall and bladder. You can see whether the baby is presenting head or breech (buttocks) first. By measuring the head, one can determine the age of the fetus and estimate the date of delivery. Sonography can also be used to detect slow fetal growth. In cases in which growth is retarded, it may be decided to deliver the baby early, especially if the condition is associated with maternal illness. Sonography may also be used to determine the placement of the placenta when placenta previa is suspected or when an amniocentesis is to be done.

Amniocentesis is a procedure that can be used to test for a variety of conditions. It has been found to be safe in more than ninety-nine percent of instances used. Again, it is a test that can be done quickly and no special preparation is needed. First, a sonogram is usually done to locate the position of the placenta and fetus. Then a thin needle is passed through the abdomen into the uterus and approximately ten millimeters of amniotic fluid is withdrawn. A local anesthetic is sometimes used, so that this causes no more pain than the average injection. If you're squeamish you might want to bring along the father for moral support, and fathers usually enjoy seeing the sonogram of the fetus.

The amniotic fluid can be used to investigate many aspects of the developing fetus. For example, it contains cells cast off from the fetus, and by growing these cells and then examining them under a microscope the chromosomes can be studied and many chromosomal abnormalities can be detected. (And of course the sex of the fetus is also apparent.) More and more doctors are recommending that amniocentesis be done for pregnant women age thirty-five or over during the first trimester. The reason is that genetic abnormalities, particularly Down's syndrome (mongolism), increase markedly among women in this age group. The test should also be performed if there is a known genetic disease in the family, such as Tay-Sachs.

The amniotic fluid can also be studied for the presence and amount of various chemicals which give indications of fetal and placental function and maturity. For women who are Rh negative and sensi-

Children love to feel a baby moving in the womb.

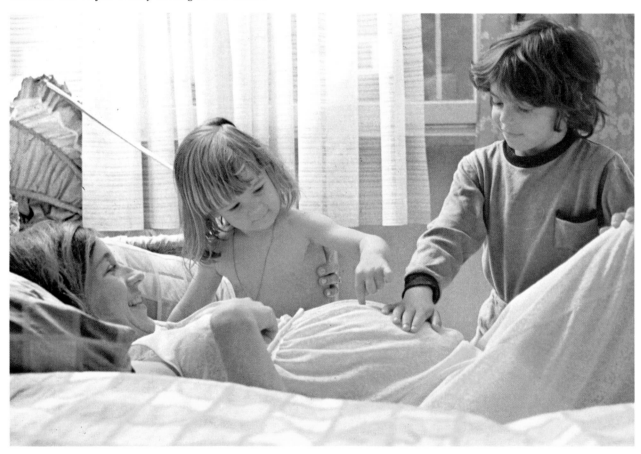

tized from previous pregnancies, amniocentesis can be used to determine fetal well-being at various times during pregnancy.

A third commonly used diagnostic technique is the analysis of the level of estriol in blood and urine samples from the mother. Estriol is an estrogen which is produced by the feto-placenta unit from chemical precursors in the mother. It's excreted by the placenta into the mother's bloodstream and eventually enters her urine. Serial measurements of estriol give an indication of fetal well-being. The test may be advised if you're past your estimated date of delivery, or if you have some known difficulty, such as diabetes or high blood pressure. If the levels of estriol fall precipitously, there may be an indication for early delivery by the induction of labor or Caesarian section.

The experience of pregnancy sets a woman apart, even in some ways from her previous self. It is a mysterious event that in a fundamental sense cannot be shared. Nevertheless, preparing for a child can be shared and this is vitally important to most pregnant women and their families. The pregnant woman who feels isolated is seldom happy. A father who feels shut out by a pregnancy, and doesn't think he has a role in the preparations for the child, may feel lonely and angry. And if there are older children in the family, they, too, need to be involved in getting ready for the baby. It may be too much to ask an older child to welcome a baby (although it does happen), but he or she is more apt to accept the situation if a realistic idea of what to expect is given. Surprises are upsetting.

One of the advantages of childbirth classes or classes in the care of newborns (which are given by many hospitals) is that fathers are included and can see that they have important responsibilities apart from paying bills. In prepared-birth classes, the father learns techniques for helping the woman with labor, and is usually present at birth. But whatever method of delivery you choose, it's best if it's a joint decision. Ideally, the father should meet your obstetrician and have a good rapport with him or her.

Traditionally, the pregnant woman and her mother or mother-in-law go shopping for the baby. This deprives the father of the fun of choosing things for his child. Shopping for a baby is one of life's very pleasant pastimes, and fathers should be involved, too.

Older children, however, often don't like shopping, especially for a new baby, and shouldn't be dragged into it. A child who picks out one gift for a new sibling has probably exhausted his generosity. An older child might better go to the movies with one of his grandparents than shopping with his parents.

It's equally important during a pregnancy for members of the family to be aware of each other's feelings, and to communicate with each other. Fathers often experience anxieties and discomforts similar to those of pregnant women, but are embarrassed to talk about them. Some men, for example, have symptoms of morning sickness, and many are frightened as the time for birth approaches. Another common reaction is jealousy of the woman for her experience of bearing a child. In some cultures, couvade rites, in which the man acts out labor and birth, provide a means of expressing and resolving these feelings. Unfortunately, our rituals for the father, such as going out drinking or handing out cigars at the office, separate him from the birth. But more fathers today feel able to empathize openly with the mother and express their concerns about the pregnancy and the baby. And as the parents share their experiences, each is better able to help the other.

Older children should be encouraged to talk about the new baby, but this doesn't mean questioning a child every day to find out if he's developing neuroses over the future sibling. There's no need to tell a young child that you're pregnant until several months have passed (unless he's going to hear it from someone else). If you wait until the baby is active, this is a good time for the announcement. Children love to feel the baby kicking, and touching her makes the baby more real and less threatening.

If an older child is going to have to change his room or bed or make other adjustments when the baby is born, try to get him started on these at least a couple of months before the baby is due. Make arrangements well ahead of time for his care when you're in the hospital. The ideal is for the father to take a few days off from work with extra help from a favorite relative or baby sitter. Unfortunately, very few hospitals allow children to visit their new brothers and sisters. Parents report that when this is allowed, there's much less upset and rivalry when the baby comes home.

An older child usually likes to be told that a baby is just a baby and can't do any of the things a big girl or boy can do. Plan to make it clear that when the baby comes home the older child gets promoted to big brother or sister. Let him stay up a half hour later at night or watch a new TV show or learn to ride a two-wheel bike. The older child will probably still want babying and reassurance for a while, but he'll feel better if he can see at least some advantages to his situation.

For many mothers, and sometimes for the whole family, the expected baby seems to become a real person even before she's born. The baby is welcomed and loved immediately. Sometimes these feelings appear in dreams, as in this one a new mother recalled for her child: "I had a wonderful dream about you. I dreamt I was standing somewhere and it was night. Suddenly a little star fell from the sky. But the star wasn't like most stars. It was you."

Labor & Birth

Waiting for labor to begin and the baby to be born, the expectant mother—and father—imagine it all a thousand times. They review over and over what has to be packed, how they'll get to the hospital, what they have to buy for the baby. A woman who hasn't had a child before tries to imagine what labor will be like, how she'll react and how she'll feel when she first sees her baby. She makes good resolutions: She'll go into labor rested and calm. She won't tense up. She won't go to the hospital too soon. And, of course, she won't go too late.

As often as not, after months of good planning, something surprising happens at the last minute. The woman goes into labor in the middle of a New Year's party when she isn't rested at all. Labor begins two weeks before it's supposed to while she's out on a boat fishing. The labor goes more quickly than she expected, or more slowly.

Are the anticipation and planning wasted? Not at all. The more knowledgeable and prepared the parents are, the better they can cope with surprises. They have found a doctor and hospital of which they're confident. They're certain that labor won't be dangerously painful or prolonged. Under these circumstances, childbirth can be an exciting and totally satisfying experience.

During the course of your pregnancy, your doctor or midwife will explain to you how to recognize the beginning of labor, when you should notify him or her that labor has started and when you should go to the hospital. The three standard signs of labor are generally considered to be regular uterine contractions, rupture of the amniotic sac (your "water breaks") and a "bloody show."

Contractions usually begin at irregular intervals and become more regular over the course of a few hours. The regularity and increasing intensity is what distinguishes true labor. Contractions typically begin as cramping sensations over the symphasis pubis, the pubic bone, the small bone low in the front of your pelvis. Early contractions may last only twenty-five to thirty-five seconds and come in an

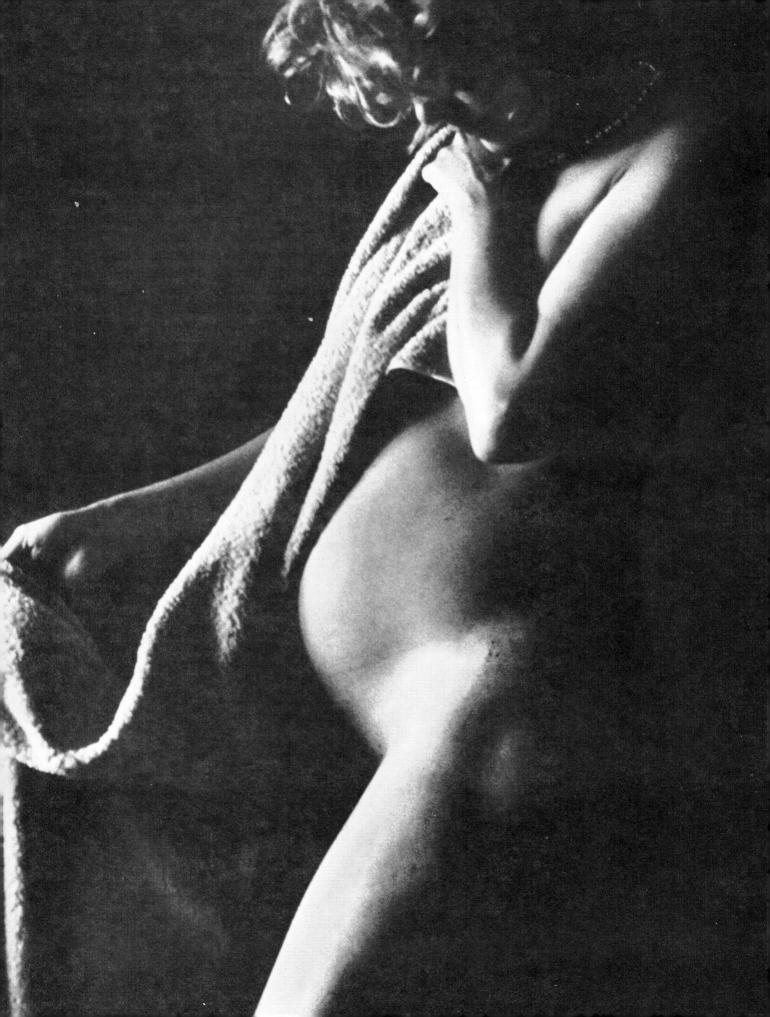

A Braxton-Hicks contraction
subtly outlines the baby whose
bottom is just in front of the
mother's elbow.

irregular pattern, from four to fifteen minutes apart. Gradually, they will establish a pattern of approximately five-minute intervals. They will also start to last longer, usually forty to sixty seconds. Their intensity will increase, and during a contraction you may feel a tight band of pressure, first in your back and then moving around to the front of the uterus. Some women experience most of labor as sharp sensations centered in the sacral area of the back. It is believed that this "back labor" is due to the force of the contractions pressing the baby's head against the mother's spinal column.

The amniotic sac may rupture before or after the onset of regular contractions. If the rupture occurs before labor starts, which happens in about twelve percent of pregnancies, you can expect that labor will begin soon, probably within twenty-four to forty-eight hours. If labor does not start spontaneously, your doctor will most likely want to induce it to minimize any chance of infection.

It's a common mistake to think that if your "water breaks" early this will result in a "dry" labor, which is said to be more painful. Actually, new fluid is continually produced by the placenta and fetus, and dryness doesn't occur.

When the amniotic membranes break, there may be a sudden gush of two to six ounces of fluid or the fluid may escape in a slow continuous trickle. The fluid is usually clear. You should note the time that your membranes rupture and the color of the fluid. If it is yellow or greenish, this is due to the presence of meconium expelled from the baby's bowels, which may indicate fetal stress. Your doctor will want to know about this, and he will try to determine if there is a significant problem and will monitor the labor carefully.

A "bloody show" is a thick mucoid discharge, colored bright red, which results from the breaking of small capillaries as the cervix dilates. It is often confused with the pink-tinged discharge that may occur near term or with the loss of the mucous plug that blocks the cervix. This plug appears as a clump of mucus in clotted brown-colored blood, and is accompanied by spots of bleeding. You may lose it as early as a few days to a week before labor, especially if you've already had a child. The "bloody show," however, usually doesn't appear until the cervix is already well dilated. Don't wait for this sign of labor before calling your doctor. The baby is already very much en route.

It isn't known exactly what triggers labor to begin, but the mechanics of the process are quite well understood.

An unborn baby is very securely sealed in place. This is perhaps even more true with humans than other mammals because we stand upright and, therefore, the pull of gravity has to be counteracted. In a pregnant woman the cervix is closed tight, sealed with the mucous plug, and sealed again by the amniotic sac containing the baby. This closed passage must be forced open for the baby to be born. Uterine contractions dilate (stretch) and efface (flatten) the cervix; they also exert downward pressure, pushing the baby's head against the cervic. This effacement and dilation of the cervix resembles what happens to the neck of a turtleneck sweater as you put your head through. The cervix, too, changes from a tubular shape to a plain circular opening. When it is ten centimeters dilated, the baby can pass into the vaginal canal.

Labor is most often a slow process, and it's not necessary to rush to the hospital when regular contractions begin. For a woman having her first baby, it usually takes about nine hours from the onset of regular contractions for the cervix to become three centimeters dilated; for a woman who has already had a child, it takes about five hours. This is the latent phase of labor. The active phase (dilation from three centimeters to ten centimeters) takes an average of five hours for a first child and two and a half hours for a successive child. And then the pushing begins. In total, a woman having her first child will probably spend about sixteen hours in labor and the woman having a successive child will probably labor about eight hours. (These figures are based on a well-known study done by Dr. M. A. Friedman, and represent a statistical pattern. Any individual's

A traditional good-bye kiss. Today, though, the husband may be joining his wife after she's settled, especially if they've studied prepared child-birth together.

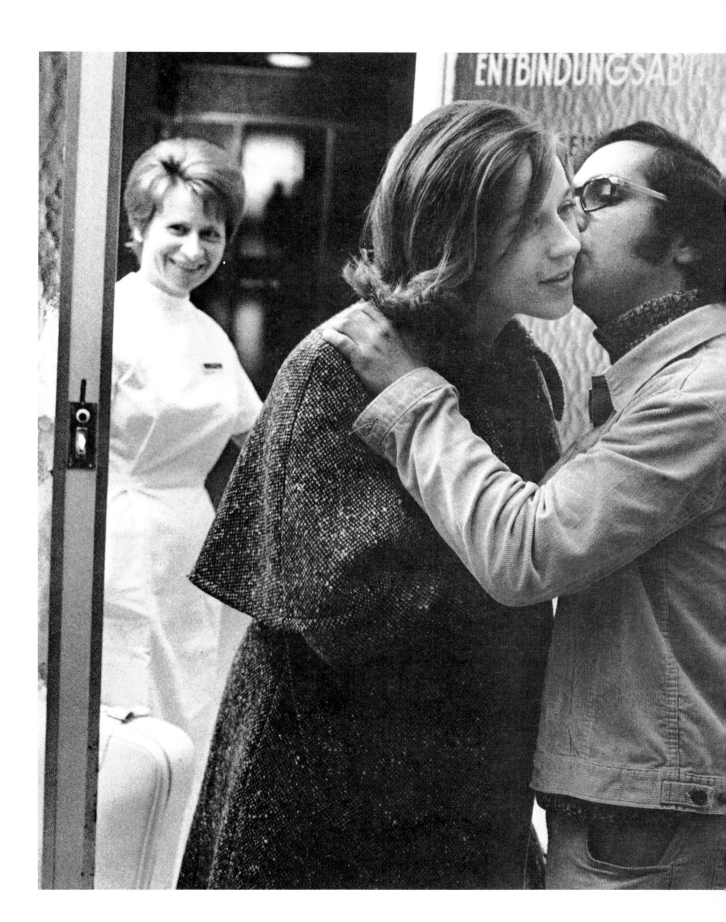

experience may vary considerably from the norm. But you're very unlikely to have your baby in an hour or two.) The most significant factors are the state of the cervix and level of the baby's presenting part when the contractions begin.

During the hours you're at home in early labor, try to keep yourself as active as possible. You may find it comfortable to take a shower and wash your hair. Be very careful getting in and out of the shower. In the British Isles and Europe, it's common practice to give baths to all women in labor when they enter the hospital but this custom is not followed in the United States because of fear of infection.

Check that your bag is packed with all the things you'll need in the hospital, including toilet articles and a nightgown and robe to wear for guests. When you're alone, you'll probably find the hospital gowns more convenient, especially at night. Why risk staining your own clothes with the vaginal discharge or breast milk? You should also bring a few sturdy bras. Even if you're not going to breast feed, you should wear a good bra twenty-four hours a day for about a week after you deliver. This well help prevent engorgement of the breasts and give the tissues support.

Items you should have ready at home but which you needn't take to the hospital include sanitary napkins and a sanitary belt. You can expect some bleeding for one to two weeks after delivery, and tampons are not used because of the risk of infection. In the hospital, sanitary pads will be provided. (The ones you have at home may also be useful if your membranes rupture early.)

Clothes for the baby are also best left at home until after you've delivered, so they don't get mislaid. For taking the baby home, you should have an undershirt and a jumpsuit or some similar outfit; there should be coverings for the baby's feet and head. Even in the summer, an infant loses a great amount of body heat from his head and extremities. You should also have a thin receiving blanket and, if the weather is cold, a heavy bunting. The hospital will usually give you a diaper for the baby and enough formula to last one or two days.

For your husband, pack some food, such as a sandwich and fruit, if he is planning to stay with you. It may be hard for him to find food at the hospital, especially good food; and he'll need a break from time to time to eat and regain his physical and emotional strength. It's not easy for a father to remain calm and cheerful throughout the labor, and then after the baby's born and the mother can sleep, he's faced with calling all the friends and relatives.

Don't eat a big meal before going to the hospital. In active labor, digestion stops. A mass of food in your stomach is no help and would be dangerous if you were to vomit. In early labor you need fluids and calories. Broth, ginger ale, tea and Jell-O are especially good, because they're easily digested. You can eat more than this if you feel comfortable, but don't take large amounts of solid food.

When you're in the hospital, you probaby won't be given water to drink, but you may be allowed to suck on ice chips or lollipops (the sour ones are best for relieving dryness—many women bring some along with them to the hospital).

Your doctor will probably want you in the hospital by the time you're about four to five centimeters dilated and the contractions are three to five minutes apart. Many hospitals encourage expectant parents to visit the labor and lying-in areas before the baby is due, so that they'll be familiar with the setup and meet some of the hospital personnel. If you're the type of person who becomes anxious in hospitals, it's a good idea to take advantage of this opportunity. The obstetrics division of a hospital is usually a happy place, even if the decor is drab. You should be made welcome when you arrive.

Before admission, you'll be taken to a labor room or curtained cubicle and asked to undress for a pelvic exam to be sure that you're in active labor. A doctor, midwife or nurse will check the dilation of

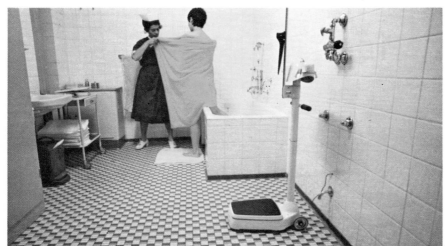

A bath is relaxing early in labor. In European hospitals women in labor are given a bath after entering the hospital.

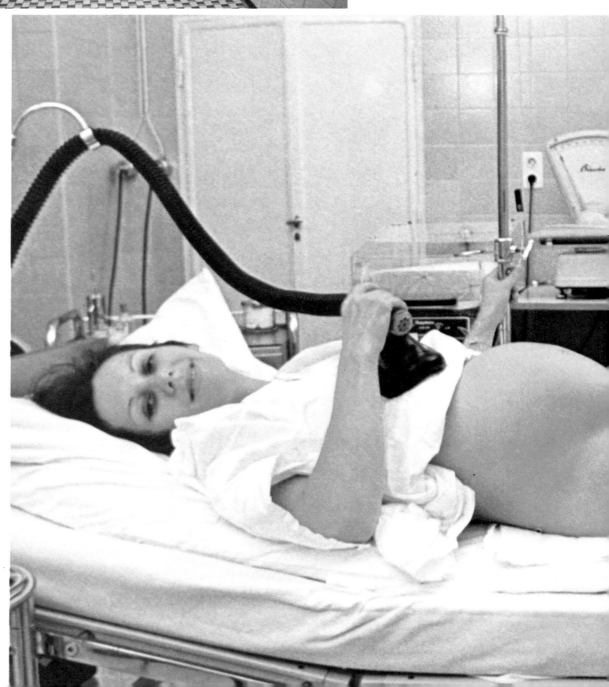

At ease and happy, a woman rests between contractions in the first stage of labor. She has nitrous oxide (laughing gas) at hand to use as she wants, which is customary in Europe. The baby will be delivered in this same room (see the scales and incubator in the background). Using one room only is an excellent arrangement that's beginning to appear in the United States, too.

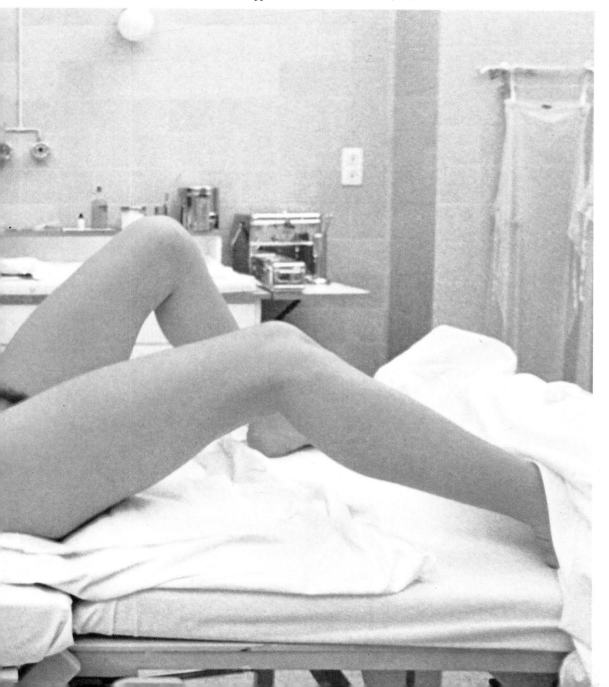

your cervix and whether the baby's head has descended into the bony structure of the pelvis. (In a breech presentation, the baby's buttocks descend first.)

If it's decided that you should be admitted to the labor floor, you'll most likely receive a shave and enema. Most doctors today request only a small shave of the area immediately surrounding the vagina; a few don't bother at all. Many doctors skip the enema, especially if the woman has had a recent bowel movement. It used to be thought that a hot enema speeded up labor, but probably the only reason that labor is stronger after an enema is that giving an enema takes time. The purpose of the enema is to cleanse the lower bowel so that feces will not be expelled as the baby's head exerts pressure on the rectum.

On admission, some blood may be drawn from a vein and an intravenous drip (an I.V.) will most likely be started. The I.V. is usually a solution of sugar and water to prevent dehydration and provide quick calories during labor and delivery. The I.V. also provides a quick route for giving medication if it's necessary.

Many doctors use Pitocin routinely in the I.V. Pitocin is a synthetic version of the hormone oxytocin, which stimulates contractions. You should certainly feel free to ask if there is any Pitocin in the I.V. and, ideally, you should already have discussed with your doctor under what circumstances he uses it. Medically it's indicated if the onset of labor is unduly delayed (for example, following the rupture of the membranes) or if labor is progressing so slowly it might be dangerous to the mother or baby. Pitocin has been used freely to accelerate labor for reasons of convenience, but it provokes contractions that are more rapid, vigorous and uncomfortable than normal. It's difficult for a woman to cope with this kind of labor without anesthetic, and the contractions have to be constantly monitored to be sure they don't become too strong for the baby to tolerate.

When you're in labor your vital signs (pulse, respiration, blood pressure) will be checked regularly. The frequency and duration of the contractions and the fetal heartbeat will also be monitored.

Most hospitals in the United States now have modern fetal monitoring equipment. These machines record the mother's contractions (showing their intensity and duration) on a sheet of graph paper, while simultaneously recording the baby's heart rate. This allows the doctor to know at all times how the baby's heart is responding to the mother's labor pattern.

There are two ways of applying these monitors. It can be done externally, with two bands attached around the woman's abdomen. One band, placed high on the abdomen (on the fundus, the top of the uterus), has a small pressure-sensitive button that responds to changes in the abdominal wall during a contraction. The other band, placed lower, picks up the baby's heartbeat. After the mother's membranes have ruptured, an internal recording device can be used. The method is painless. During a pelvic exam, a thin wire is attached to the top of the baby's head (or to his buttocks), which transmits the heartbeat. At the same time, a thin tube can be threaded up into the uterus, which records the pressure exerted with each contraction. Believe it or not, this causes no discomfort—you shouldn't even feel it. Many women prefer this internal method because it's less annoying than bands around the abdomen. It's also more accurate.

Fetal monitoring machines are invaluable for detecting potential problems before they become serious. Some doctors feel they should be used in every labor. They are also compatible with "natural" childbirth methods. Some women find that the bands interfere somewhat with the exercises; but, on the positive side, the machine can help a woman time her breathing, because a labor nurse or coach can see the beginning of a contraction, often before the woman herself can feel it, and can warn her to start her breathing exercise. The coach can also see when a contraction has peaked and is starting to ebb, which can be encouraging news to the mother.

Labor rooms are often rather grim and dull, containing one or

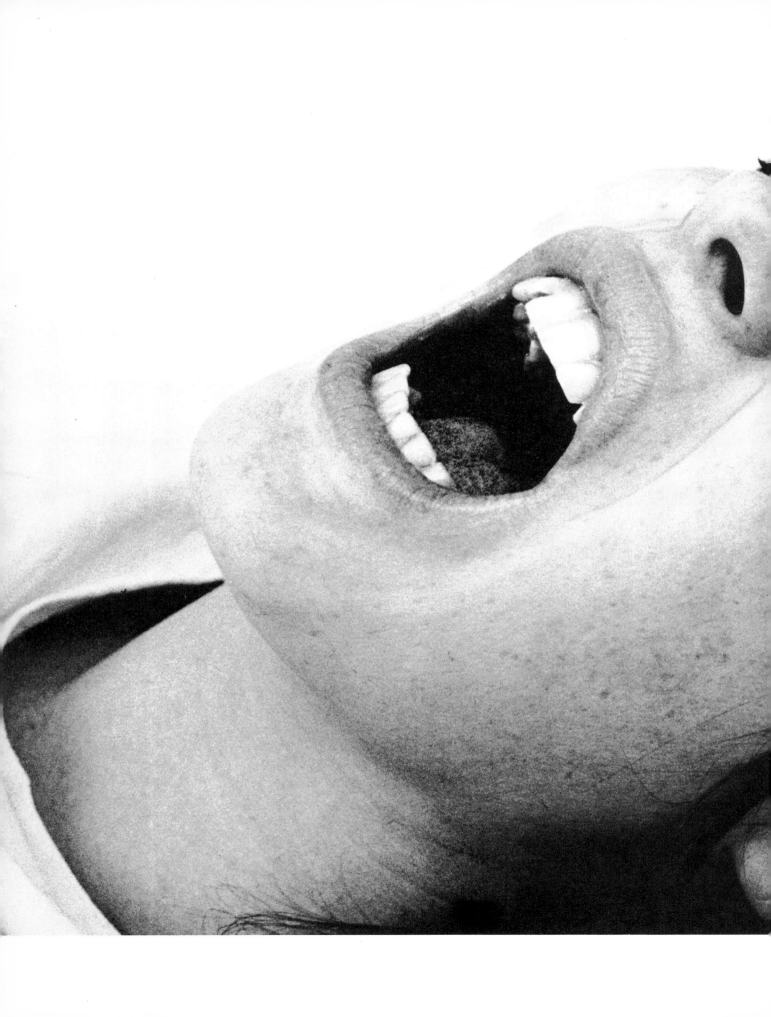

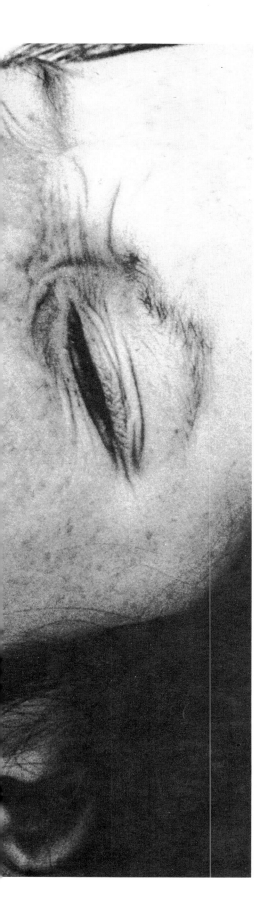

two labor beds, one or two chairs and possibly a bedside table. There are usually also a blood-pressure cuff, various stethoscopes, I.V. equipment and the like. Undoubtedly, in the future, these rooms will become more attractive and homelike as more and more women look for a pleasanter environment for having a baby. This concern isn't simply frivolous. Uncomfortable furnishings and an institutional ambience tend to make people tense and tired.

Labor floors are generally extremely active at all times of the day and night. You may see midwives, nurses and nursing assistants, doctors and medical students, clerks and orderlies, women in labor and their husbands. With you will perhaps be your husband and your personal labor coach, if you've arranged for one (most often done through prepared-birth classes). All the comings and goings can be confusing. It may help to ask exactly who each person is who comes into your room. Your labor nurse will probably be your best source of information and guidance.

Toward the end of the first stage of labor, most women find they're working hard. Some feel they can't keep up with the labor, that they're being overwhelmed. This is when encouragement and possibly a tranquilizer and analgesic, such as Demerol, can be helpful. Perhaps the most difficult time is during the "transition," at the end of the first stage of labor. The cervix is almost fully dilated and the baby's head is being pushed through it. Contractions come every two to three minutes and last close to a minute. The mother may experience general malaise, nausea and trembling of her limbs. She may also feel a strong urge to begin pushing the baby out by holding her breath and bearing down with her abdominal muscles. But if she's not yet fully dilated, the pushing may cause the cervix to swell or even tear. She's told to hold back; not to push, but to blow out instead. This is difficult and uncomfortable, but within a few minutes to an hour, the cervix will be fully dilated and pushing can begin.

During the second stage of labor, the mother is pushing the baby

A mother is wheeled into a de-livery room (which is lighter and brighter than most). Note the baby scales, gas dispenser (at left), sterilizing equipment.

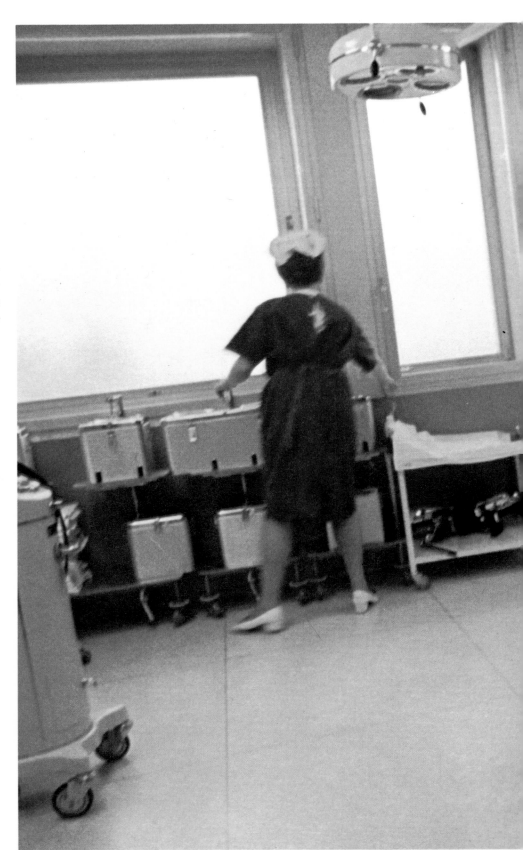

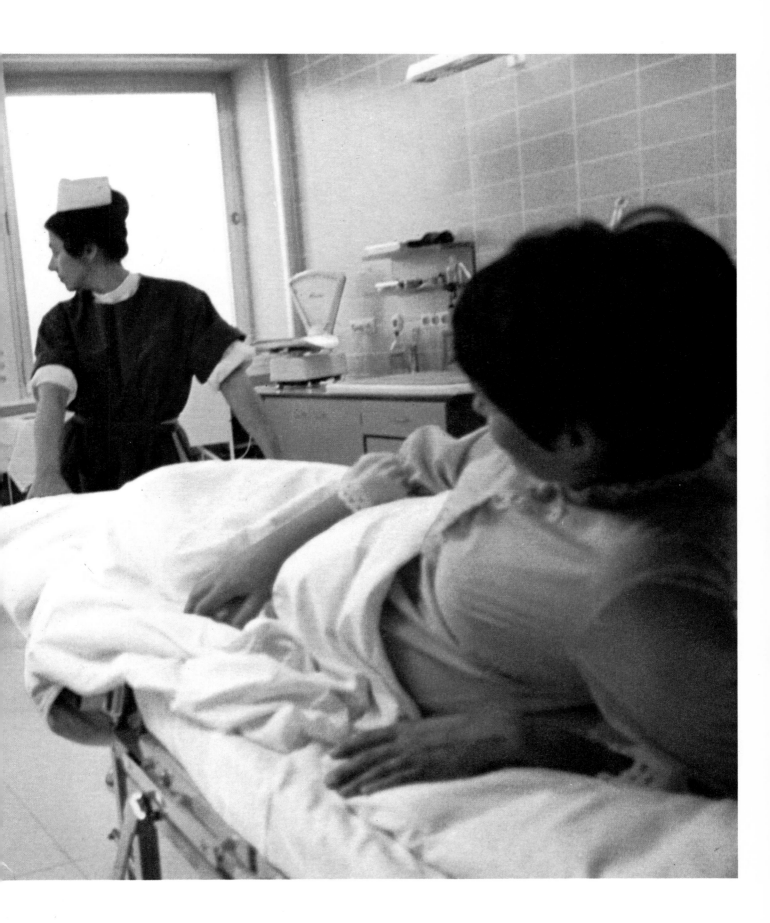

out of the vagina. Contractions come about two to three minutes apart, and the urge to bear down is very strong. This stage usually lasts about an hour with a first baby and thirty to forty minutes with a successive child. During this time the mother may feel out of herself, as if swept away by the force of giving birth. She is working very hard, perhaps harder than ever before in her life (but often the discomfort is less than in the previous stage).

You'll be wheeled into the delivery room when the baby's head can be seen at the vaginal opening, about ten minutes before the baby is expected. (Some hospitals now have rooms in which both labor and delivery can be managed, which is a marvelous convenience.) The delivery table has stirrups and supports for your feet and legs. You'll be covered with sterile sheets that have an opening between your legs. There may be straps for tying your arms so that you don't inadvertently touch the sterile area around your genitals. But this strapping is done in fewer and fewer hospitals now that women have started demanding more sympathetic and dignified treatment in childbirth. It's something you can and should discuss ahead of time with your doctor.

There will be equipment for giving gas, if it's needed, and a mirror so that you and the father (if he's there) can see the baby being born. There will also be equipment for stimulating the baby's breathing if it doesn't start spontaneously.

A delivery room can seem crowded with people and sometimes is. In addition to your doctor, there may be an anesthetist, a nurse, perhaps a midwife, and a pediatrician. You can ask your doctor to explain who will be present. You have the right to as much privacy as is consistent with good medical care.

The birth of the baby concludes the second stage of labor, the third being the expulsion of the placenta, or afterbirth, usually minutes later.

When you first hear and see your baby, you may feel the most profound longing to hold and protect her, while the doctors and nurses are trying to whisk her away to the nursery. Recently, a number of doctors, including Dr. Marshall Klaus and Dr. Lee Salk, have emphasized that this is a natural and important reaction, and parents shouldn't be treated as if they were hysterical because they want to hold their own child. However, it *is* essential that the baby's heartbeat, respiration and general physical condition be checked. If you're not overtired, you'll probably be allowed to spend some time with the baby. And you can ask to have her brought to you at the next feeding time if you're awake and ready to hold her.

The experience of labor and birth transcends the physiology of the event. Often women feel they can't find the words to describe it. But their first-hand accounts always convey a sense of drama and excitement. These are the reactions of some of the women interviewed for this book:

"At first I only felt a very fine twinging in my back. Half curious, half fearful, I listened to myself. Then all at once, I knew: It's starting. I felt lonesome, weak and abandoned. At the same time, I was filled with a grave feeling, both earnest and holy at once. In the delivery room, the contractions washed over me like irresistible waves. I imagined I was in an ocean. I allowed myself to drift in a wide swell. Up and down. Back and forth. I was part of nature. I thought a great deal about myself during the hours of the opening phase; I thought about my life, my mother, my husband, and naturally, my child, who was trying to come out. The labor pains lasted for seven hours. There were so many times I wanted to give up! But I managed to hold on. Afterward, all the troubles are forgotten. The strain is worth it."

"In the opening phase, the labor pains were stormy gusts. Then I was flung into a typhoon, and I felt as if I were whirling through the air. 'Don't push,' I kept hearing the midwife say. But I felt something like an incredible need to move my bowels. I just couldn't hold back. There was a terrific weight on my pelvis, and it kept growing and growing. 'I just can't help it,'

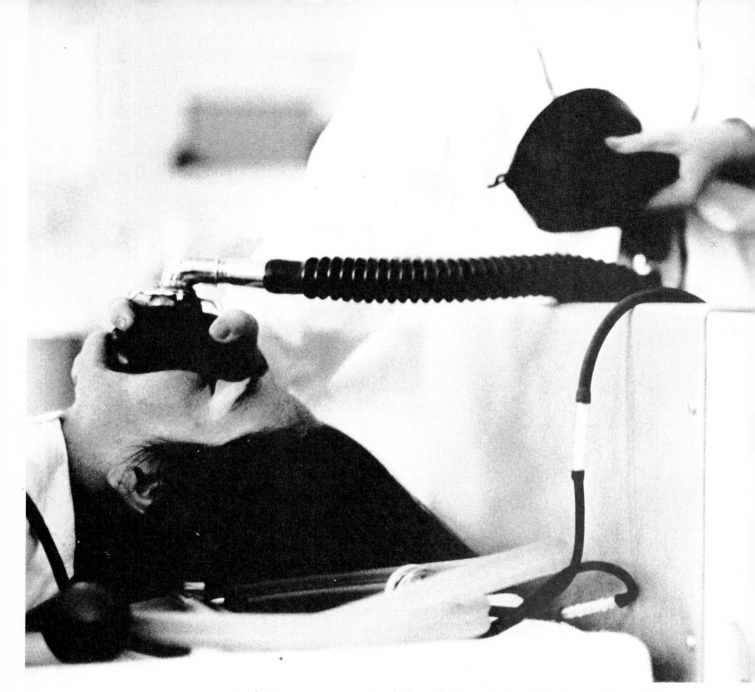

In the past, women were given full anesthesia as the time of birth nears. Here, while the baby is being delivered, the anesthetist pumps the anesthesia bag rhythmically to assist the mother's breathing.

I screamed. All I wanted to do was push. I just had to squeeze that unbearable weight out of me. Just push, push, push. I had to use my last bit of strength. It's a good thing nature doesn't leave you any choice. It was an intoxication of unbelievable fatigue and volcanic eruption. Ever since I went through that experience, I know what a powerful force life is."

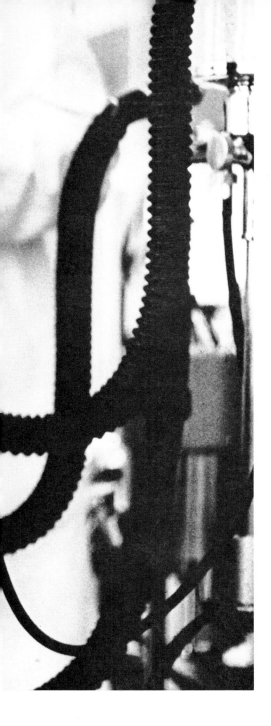

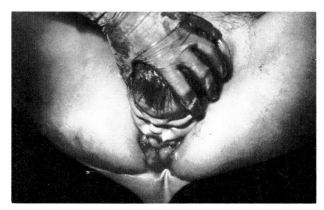

A hand on the baby's head guides its birth.

49

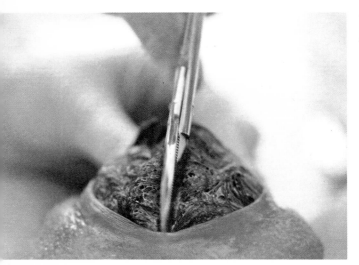

The episiotomy is a small incision in the perineum done to speed the passage of the baby's head and prevent tearing of the mother's tissues.

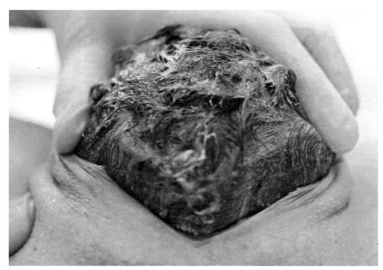

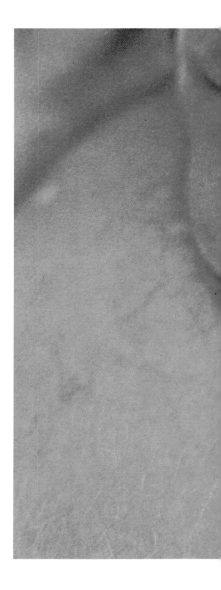

"I don't know how long the last stage of the birth lasted. In reality, it was probably only a few minutes. But it seemed like an eternity. At any rate, it lasted too long as far as I'm concerned. I yearned for a pause, just to rest up a bit and regain my strength. But a relentless force was commanding me. Like a tired, broken-down horse, I felt as if someone were whipping me along every time I threatened to falter. The expulsion pains overcame me five—or was it six—times. Even though I gave it all my strength, I felt as if nothing was moving. Why wasn't the child out yet? I was disappointed and worn out. The midwife said, 'The head's already coming!' I didn't believe a word of it."

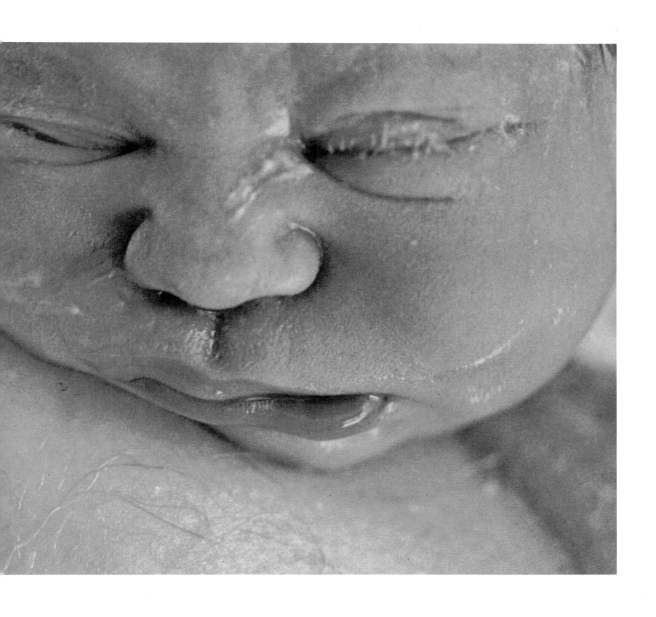

"Did I think about my child during the delivery? Yes! In my imagination, I felt as if my little baby were twisting through the narrow tunnel all by himself. It was as if I could really feel his movements. This gave me a strength I didn't realize I had: 'Just struggle along, little baby. I'll help you as much as I can. We'll make it together. I won't leave you.' That was more or less the way I was talking with my as yet unborn child. He became my partner. We were mutually dependent. Through foggy walls, I heard someone say: 'The head's all out. The worst is over.' My baby had done his work well."

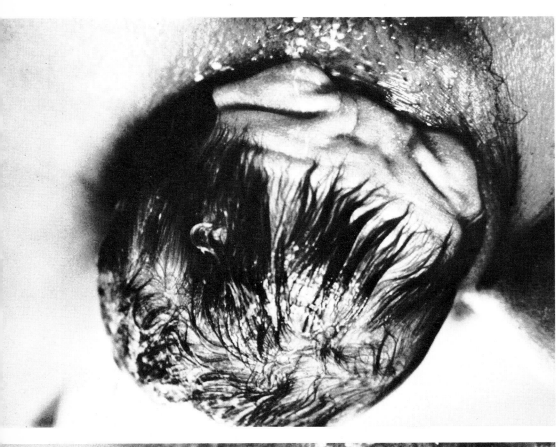

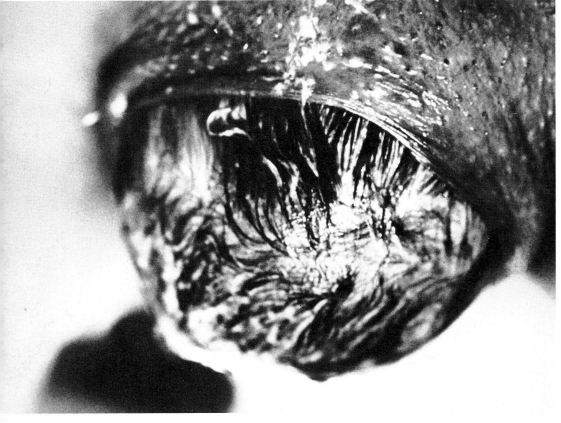

Birth is a hard experience for the baby, too. (No episiotomy has been done here.)

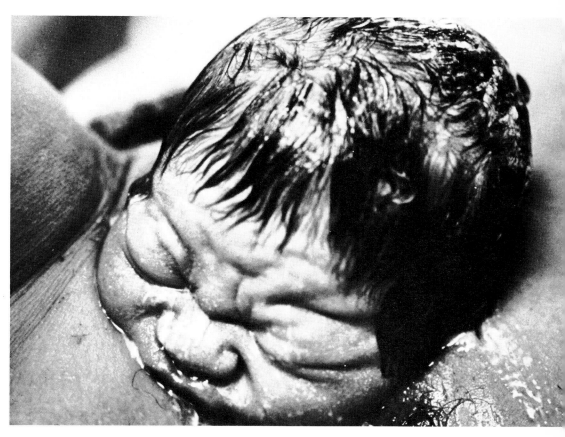

As the head emerges, it turns to one side or the other. Now the shoulders can be born, first the upper one then the lower one.

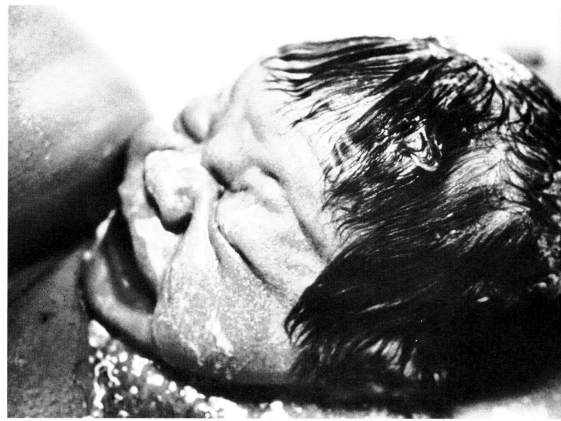

53

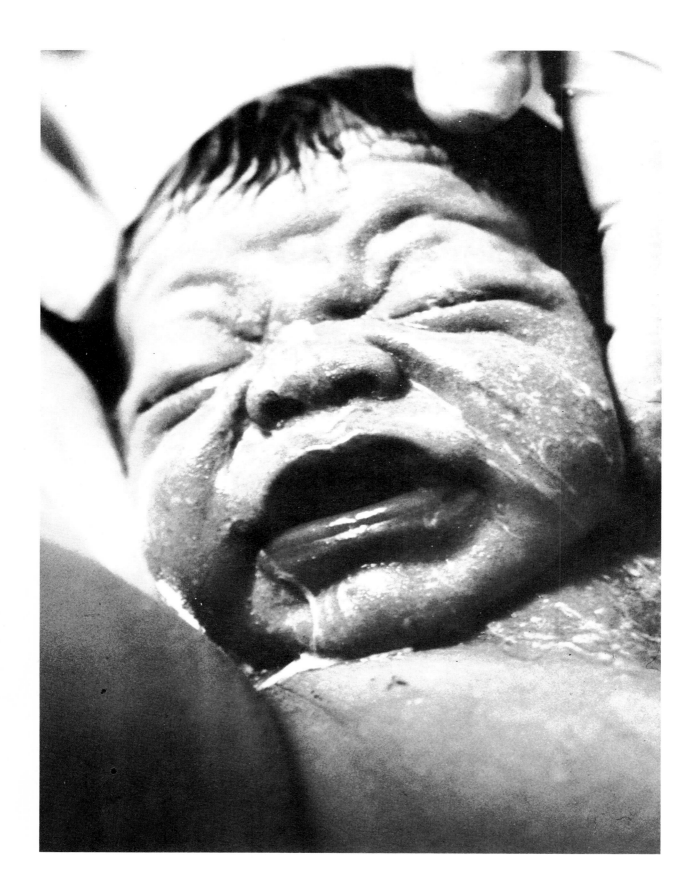

Gently, the doctor eases out the baby.

"When the head was born, the rest practically came by itself. I fell back from leaning forward in my pushing position. And while sinking back, I saw the doctor's hands between my thighs. I could make out the little head between the fingers of the gloves. A bit of damp, clinging hair. Bluish skin. Blood, there was blood too [from the episiotomy]. It glistened red and pink. A white grease [vernix]. The shoulders slipped out. Oh, what narrow, sweet shoulders! My eyes closed. I was so tired, so worn out. Whatever was happening between my legs suddenly moved far away from me. I was lying there, and somewhere else the child was climbing out. I felt separated from the birth. It was taking place without my help, after all. I drifted in an aura of unconsciousness, but without losing consciousness. The outer world vanished. I couldn't hear anything. I floated somewhere beyond space and time."

"The delivery room was silent. The midwife, the doctor or a nurse—somebody was always with me. I felt secure. It may sound conceited, but during the long opening phase I enjoyed being the center of attention. During the expulsion, with the assault-like pangs, I was much more outside of myself. I was seized by a wild force and no longer belonged to myself at all. During the final stages of the birth, everybody was interested only in the child. I must confess I felt totally lost. Just when I was about to fight harder than at any time in my life, no one helped me. Everyone was worried about the child, I received only a few terse orders. It wasn't easy for me to accept the fact that my child was suddenly becoming an independent person and that I had to give her priority for a while. It's not so easy to separate from someone. However, I don't want it to sound as if I was offended throughout the delivery, or envious, or jealous. During a birth, all kinds of feelings swirl together. In the tumult, I also had moments of self-pity, fury and protest. There was no time to collect my thoughts. My very deep experience of birth was instantly overshadowed by a radiant feeling of happiness: I've given birth to my child, and now she's here!"

55

" 'A fine healthy boy. Your baby's a boy,' said the midwife and laughed. That very instant I already heard him screaming—pretty loud for such a tiny tot. At first, I was terrified, because my child had such a blue-violet color. Was there something wrong with my child? A heart defect maybe? Was it alive? Questions like that shot through my mind. Thank goodness the blue color vanished from his complexion and gave way to a blissful pink. During

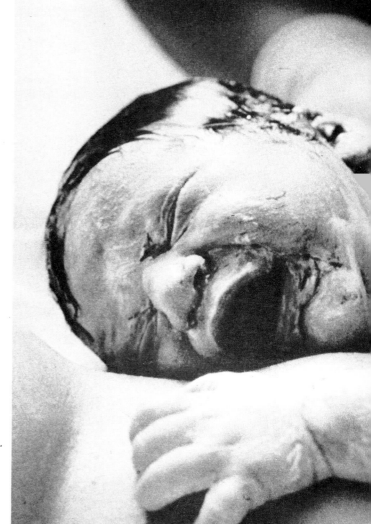

Still covered with vernix, the baby lies on her mother's stomach.

my pregnancy, my husband and I had asked thousands of times: Will it be a girl or a boy? But when our baby was born, this question didn't matter at all. As long as it was healthy! Please, just let it be healthy! And now I finally knew. I had them tell it to me ten times. A healthy, strong boy! I was so relieved, so grateful."

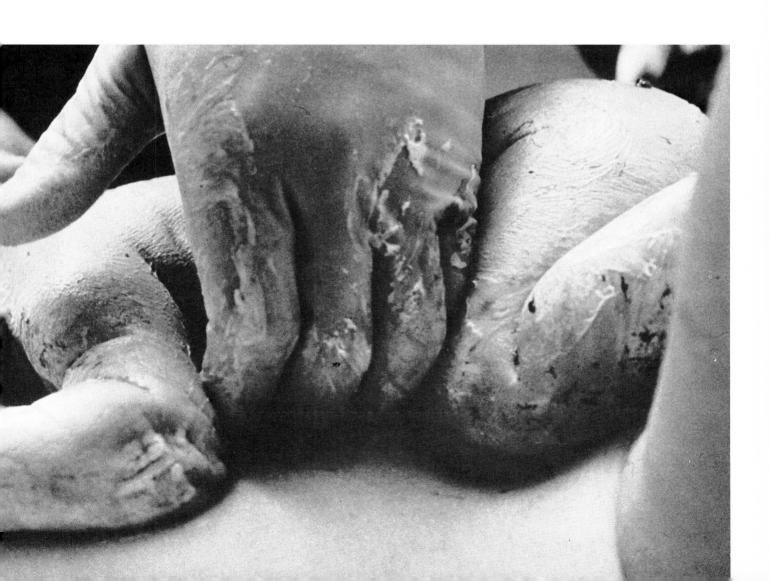

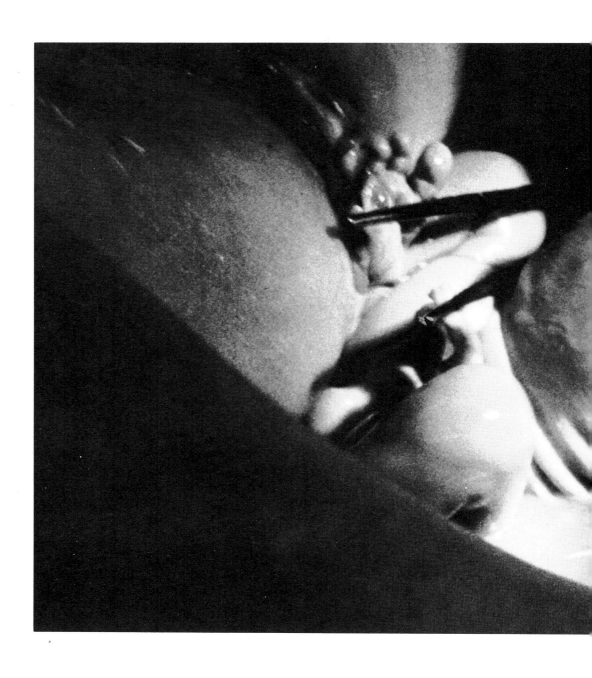

"When the doctor cut through the umbilical cord, I didn't feel anything. I just lay there, completely drained. Infinitely tired—and happy. I saw the child being carried away. My little boy was bawling. But it didn't alarm me. I was so weak I couldn't even turn my head on its side. When the midwife pressed my abdomen energetically to speed up the afterbirth, that was the last pain, like a pang. Then when they were about to sew up the episiotomy, the anesthesia carried me into the thick veils of unconsciousness. I drifted out of the depths. There were voices. There was light. And there was my child already! The midwife handed me the darling bundle. That was how my son looked—a sweet child with a worried face."

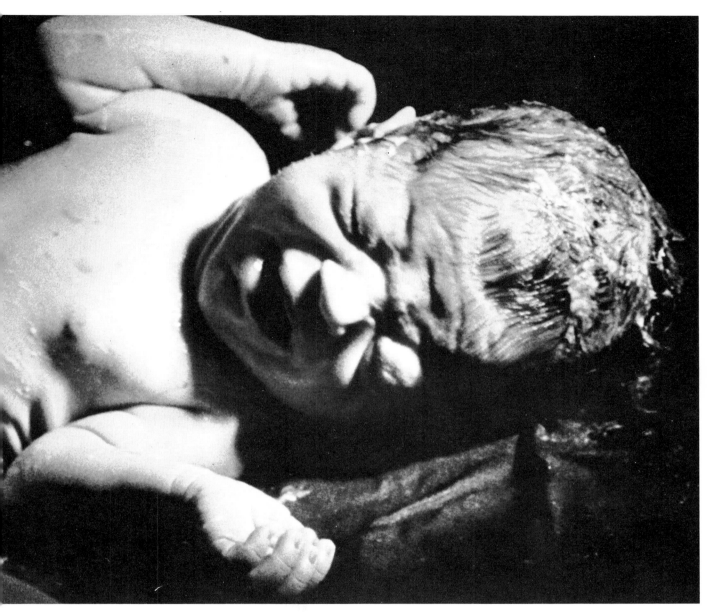

She doesn't get much of a rest yet. She's wiped off and the umbilical cord is clamped prior to cutting.

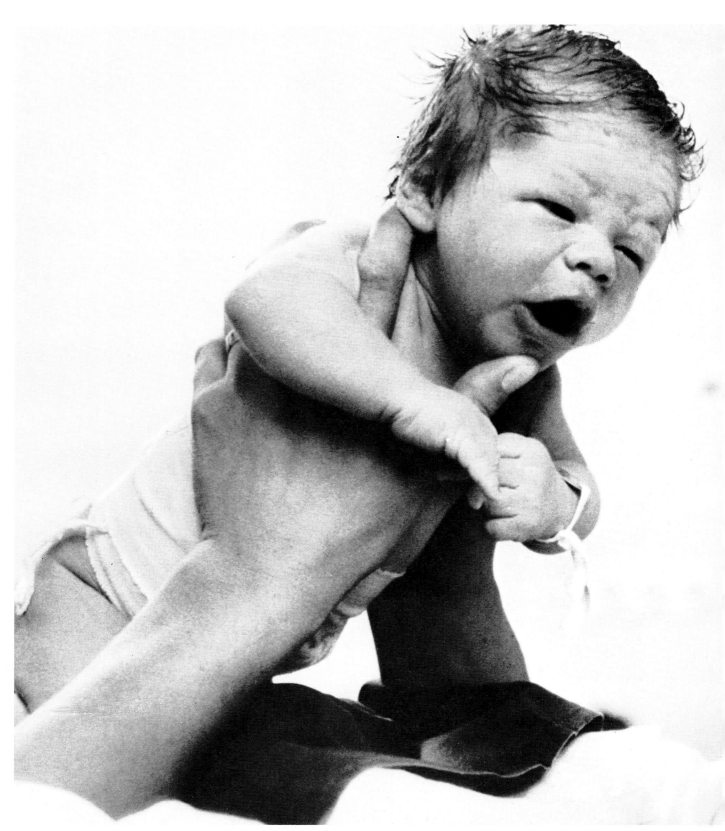

Her mother thinks she's beautiful, and soon she will be. At twelve months, she's just about perfect (see inset).

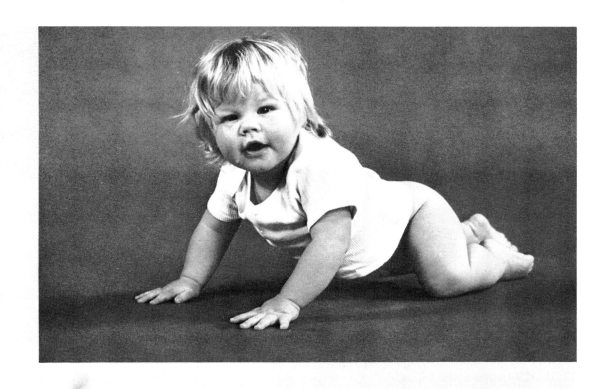

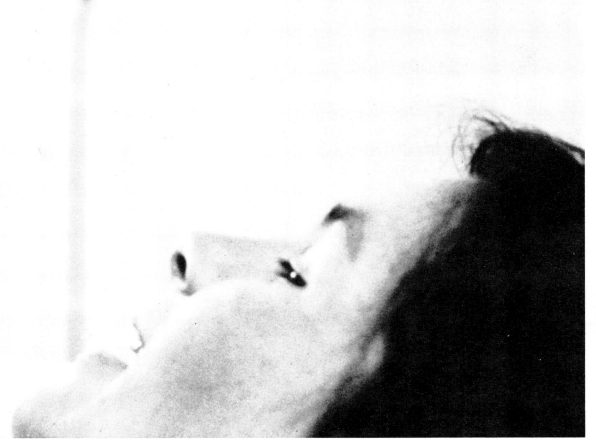

When women describe labor, as they have here, pain is not necessarily a dominant factor in their memories. Some of these women undoubtedly made use of nitrous oxide (laughing gas), which is commonly available to women in labor in England and Europe; the woman can take it when she feels the need; if she takes more than enough, she starts to lose consciousness and the gas mask drops from her hand.

Some women, however, go all the way through labor without ever asking for a painkiller. They aren't necessarily Spartan. They just don't have pain that severe.

The amount of pain women experience in labor is extremely variable. Some labors are physically more difficult than others. Some are so quick and easy the mother isn't even very tired afterward. We do know that certain subjective factors aggravate the experience of pain: fear, fatigue, tension, a feeling of being alone or abandoned and, simply, the strangeness of a first childbirth. Contractions that aren't actually painful are nevertheless unsettling and uncomfortable if they've never been experienced before. The stress can be frightening, and fear leads to pain.

Today, we are probably less well prepared to cope with pain than earlier generations were. We have such effective methods of deadening pain that it's no longer an inevitable part of life, and many of us have never dealt with severe, prolonged pain. And, in fact, why should a woman go through pain in childbirth when we have the means to free her completely from it?

Unfortunately, pain-killing substances may reduce the activity of the contractions and extend the length of labor. Even the best techniques for reducing pain are not fully free of risk, either for the mother or (especially) for the child. At term, every medication received by the mother passes across the placenta to the baby. Most women spend nine months avoiding unnecessary drugs. Certainly, then, drugs shouldn't be used carelessly in labor when they may depress the responses of the infant in the first minutes of life. This doesn't mean women shouldn't have relief from pain. But it does explain why good doctors are cautious—and why so many women study a method of prepared birth that will help them overcome discomfort.

Doctors generally prescribe limited amounts of analgesics early in labor, and reserve the more complete methods of pain relief for extreme cases of distress or later in labor. If you and your doctor or midwife talk over this issue beforehand and are in general agreement about the use of drugs, there should be no problem while you're in the hospital. If your doctor recommends medication, when you'd been hoping to do without, don't feel depressed or guilty. It's important that you be able to cooperate in the labor. If you can no longer respond to instructions or encouragement or if you become dangerously exhausted, relief is needed.

The goal in obstetrics is to balance the needs of the mother and those of the baby so that both benefit. This can be difficult, because a newborn doesn't have an adult's tolerance of drugs and cannot metabolize them as well. Overdosed babies may be born sleepy and lazy—"sleepy babies," in hospital lingo. They may not be interested in eating for days, and they have to be watched to be sure they remember to breathe. On the other hand, there's no need to allow agonizing labors that are terrible for the mother and that interfere with the smooth delivery of the child. With good use of modern techniques, you can look forward to being awake when your baby is born, and she should be awake and strong, too.

Pain relief during labor is accomplished with two broad categories of medication: analgesia, which decreases the awareness of pain; and anesthesia, which completely eliminates pain. Sedatives, such as mild tranquilizers and barbiturates, may be used as relaxing agents in early labor. They are given either orally or by intramuscular injection, and (when used early) they have usually been metabolized before the critical minutes when the baby is born. Since early contractions usually come about five or more minutes apart and don't last longer than thirty seconds, most of the pain attributed to them is the result of nervous tension, which is understandably at a peak after one has waited so long for this particular day. The relaxing action of a sedative may even allow the woman to doze off for a while.

Narcotic drugs such as Demerol (the trade name for meperidine) or morphine are generally not prescribed this early in labor because they tend to decrease contractions if a pattern has not been well established. These analgesic drugs act directly on the central nervous system. The woman remains awake and conscious but doesn't feel the contractions as intensely. Narcotics are useful later in labor; if you're having contractions that last forty-five to sixty seconds every two to three minutes, a narcotic can bring welcome relief, by decreasing their intensity and providing an interlude in which to regain your strength and composure.

Narcotic medicines are most often given either by intramuscular injection (in the hip or buttock) or in an I.V. If you have an injection, you'll feel the effect in about ten to fifteen minutes, and it will last a maximum of 1½ hours. If the drug is injected into a vein through the I.V., the effect is immediate and may be sensed as a sudden flush or "rush"; it lasts about forty-five minutes. Demerol makes some women feel dizzy or high, as if they'd had a drink or two before dinner. A fairly frequent, but passing, side effect may be nausea and vomiting. Don't be embarrassed if you become sick to your stomach. Your nurse expects this and is ready to take care of you, and the nausea usually ends very quickly.

Demerol in sizable doses can be given very late in labor, but it may depress the newborn's respiration. Should this occur there are narcotic antagonists that will reverse this depression.

In the past, large doses of Demerol were frequently combined with Scopolamine to produce a "twilight sleep." Scopolamine is an alkaloid with consciousness-altering effects. It also causes amnesia, which was considered to be a benefit. In fact, in twilight sleep, the laboring woman is often far from free of all discomfort. The medication often even provokes irritability and excitement. But because of the amnesia, mothers seldom complained. The high doses of Demerol used also affected the baby, but with the mother unable to recall her experience and the father most definitely not present at the time of delivery, the parents never knew what had happened or why junior was a "sleepy baby" and "poor feeder" for the first few days of life. This method of pain relief has appropriately fallen into disfavor, largely due to the increased knowledge of parents themselves.

Regional anesthesia causes loss of sensation in a limited area of the body without loss of consciousness. The types used most frequently in labor are local and pudendal anesthesia and paracervical, epidural and caudal blocks (the last is sometimes called a "saddle block").

The paracervical block is the easiest to administer, and can be given by either your doctor or midwife. The anesthetic agent is administered via a long needle directly around the cervix. For this you may be propped up at the end of the bed to make it easier to guide the needle into place—care must be taken that the medication isn't accidentally injected into the baby. Since the pelvic area is so copiously supplied with large blood vessels, the medicine is rapidly absorbed by the mother. It also passes across the placenta to the baby, and may cause a drop in the fetal heart rate. (This may also be caused indirectly by a brief lowering of the mother's blood pressure.)

A paracervical block lasts approximately forty-five minutes to an hour. In some situations it may be repeated, but the baby's response has to be carefully considered. Typically, this anesthesia is used to relieve the pain of cervical dilation, and, later, if the anesthesia has worn off a bit by the pushing stage, the woman has enough sensation to actively push out the baby.

Epidural and caudal anesthesia must be given by an anesthesiologist or trained obstetrician. You will be required to stay completely still, either lying on your side or sitting on the edge of the bed, with your back rounded. If you're afraid you'll move, your nurse

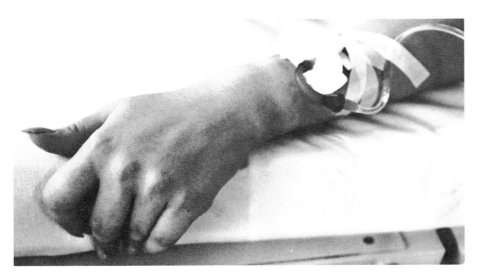

And it flows immediately into the mother's bloodstream.

With epidural anesthetic, the mother is completely conscious when her baby is born.

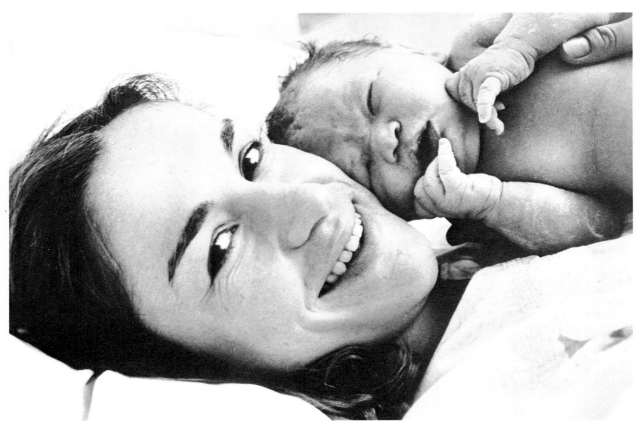

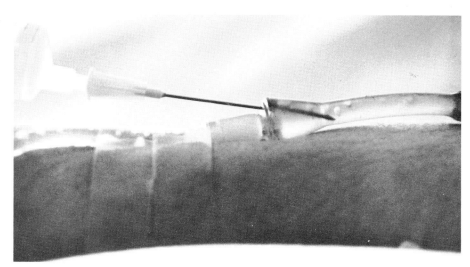

Medication can be injected directly into the I.V. solution.

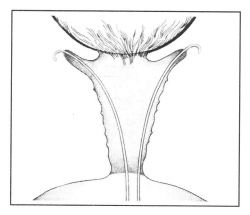

A paracervical block deadens sensation in the cervix and lower part of the uterus. The injections are made at the points shown by the arrows.

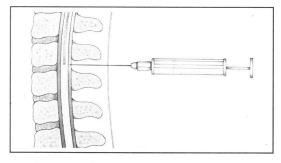

Epidural anesthesia is injected through the vertebrae, into the space between the spinal membranes.

will help hold you. When your back is curved this way, the spaces between the vertebrae of the spine are expanded. The person giving the anesthetic uses a needle through which a thin plastic tube can be passed; if it is felt that repeated doses of the medicine may be necessary, the tube is left in place. The anesthetic agent is injected into the epidural region of the spinal column; or if it is a caudal, it is given at the base of the spine. Injections of anesthetic agents directly into the central canal of the spinal column are called spinal anesthesia. Spinal anesthesia is less popular and may be associated with headaches and leave the woman completely unable to move her legs or help in pushing out the baby.

Many women, however, find that the last phase of pushing out the baby is easier than active labor while the cervix is dilating. Once they get past the transition and into pushing, they don't need the anesthetic as much, and they'd prefer to go on and push out the baby.

An epidural can be given for relief earlier in labor and, with good timing, will wear off so the woman can participate in the pushing stage of labor. If the anesthetic agent has not worn off, forceps often have to be used. Another advantage of epidural anesthesia is that it can be used for Caesarian section.

With these regional anesthetics, the woman is conscious at the birth of her baby; this is their great advantage. They are not entirely risk-free however; no anesthetic is. They have to be administered with great skill and care. But, for many women, they make the difference between a traumatic experience and a joyful one. And for many others, knowing that this relief is available if they want it reduces their fear and makes the process easier. A woman may decide to see if she can do without anesthesia for a half hour, and then another half hour, and then the baby is suddenly on his way.

If you have not had any other type of anesthesia, you will be given a local anesthetic at the time of delivery if an episiotomy is to be done. This is an incision of one to two inches made in the perineum, from the vagina toward the rectum. Local infiltration may be done to

68

deaden the nerves on the skin surface and superficial muscles of the perineum. This is done by injection with an anesthetic agent, and the area remains numb for thirty- to forty-five minutes, so there's no discomfort while the incision is being repaired. Or a pudendal block may be done by injecting anesthetic around the pudendal nerve, which is located beneath the ischial spines of the pelvic bones. This results in a more extensive area of numbness. Both methods have virtually no effect on the baby and only cause reactions in women who are allergic to "-caine" type drugs.

Nitrous oxide, or laughing gas, is a colorless, odorless gas that has an intoxicating effect. Almost every delivery room has an inhalation apparatus with a steel bottle for laughing gas and another for oxygen; the gases are mixed, and stream through a tube to a rubber mask. Nitrous oxide is used primarily to deaden the pain of the last few contractions before the baby is born or for a simple forceps delivery. The effect doesn't last very long, since the gas is excreted from the bloodstream by the lungs, and therefore, the baby is only minimally affected. The gas is safe, making you temporarily fuzzy but not unconscious.

It's impossible to decide definitely ahead of time whether medication will or won't be helpful in your labor, or which one will be most appropriate. There are numerous variables that are important, including how long you've been in labor, how long it will probably continue and, most important, how the baby is responding. You and your doctor or midwife should work as a team, with mutual aims but a flexible attitude.

Labor and childbirth are so absorbing, using all a woman's strength, that when it's over you may find you still have questions about what happened, particularly about what the medical people were doing. In fact, many of the reforms in modern obstetrics involve reducing intervention in the woman's conduct of her own labor. The first responsibility of the doctor and other medical people

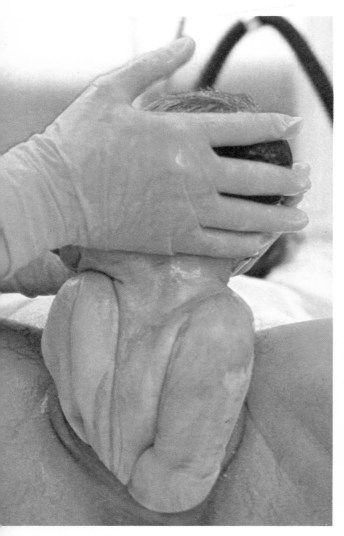

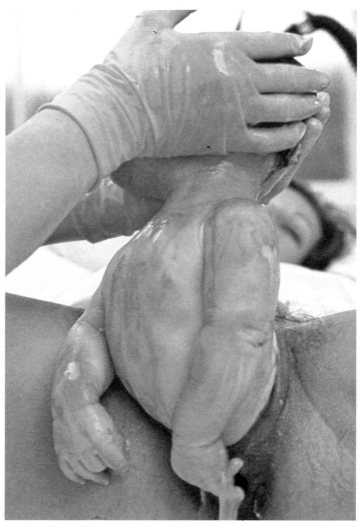

Holding the baby's head firmly, the midwife coaxes out the shoulders.

A few seconds later, the little arms are free.

is to determine whether nature is taking its usual course or whether a problem exists.

Once the process of labor has begun, it should continue at a steady, progressive rate. Your doctor needs to be sure that your cervix is dilating at a steady rate and so will perform periodic pelvic examinations. If it is not, it could mean that the uterine muscle is "tired" and may need stimulation with Pitocin. Or it could mean that the baby is too large for the pelvic opening and a Caesarian section will be needed.

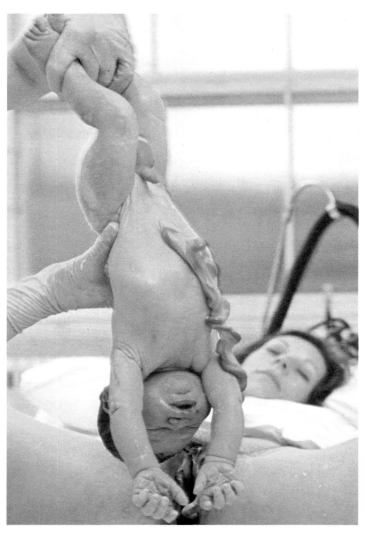

A new person is in the world.

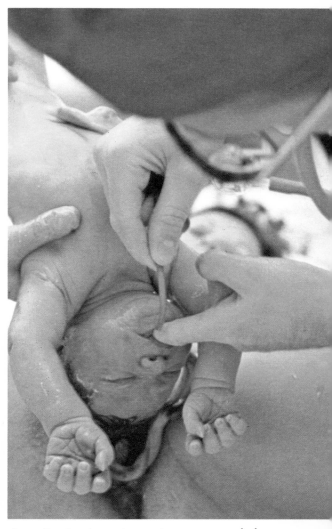

Immediately, the respiratory passages are sucked clear. The bluish tinge to the baby's hands may last for a few days.

The regular check on the vital signs of the mother and the baby's heartbeat is essential not only as a safeguard but for deciding what kind of medication if any should be given and when.

Another critical point, from the doctor's or midwife's perspective, is the moment when the woman should start pushing. They will be extremely concerned that you don't push before the cervix is fully dilated or the cervix will tear, which results not only in profuse bleeding but often in chronic irritation and infection.

During the delivery of the baby, the doctor or midwife in charge

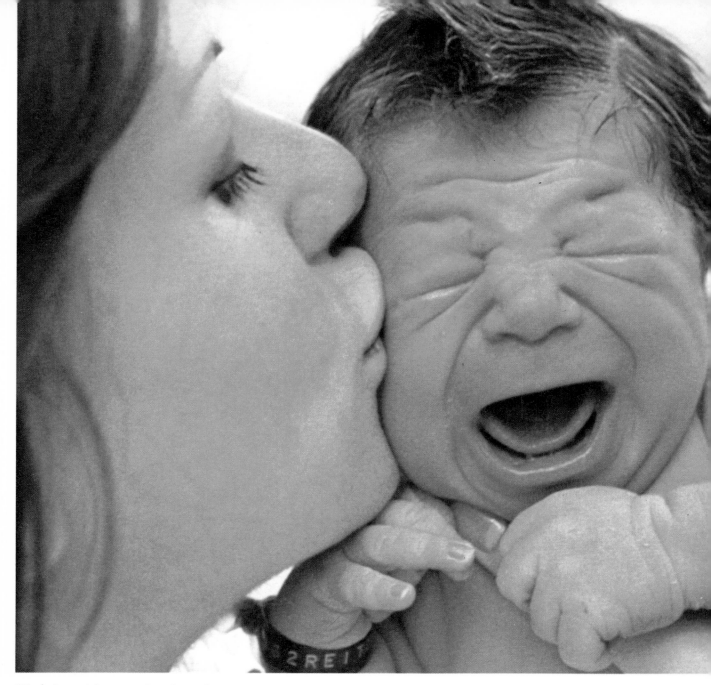

*Washed up with a name bracelet and a part in
his hair, the young man clings to his mother's
thumb while enduring his first kiss.*

is striving for a controlled delivery of the head and shoulders. This is
a critical time for the baby. Once the leading part of the baby has en-
tered the birth canal, there must be a progressive descent; otherwise
it would be a risk for both mother and child. (During the entire expulsion stage of labor, the baby's heartbeat is regularly checked to be
sure he's getting enough oxygen.) On the other hand, a too rapid delivery can be a shock to the structure of the baby's skull, which has
been compressed during the descent through the pelvic opening and
the vagina. (Most babies are born with an elongation of the head,

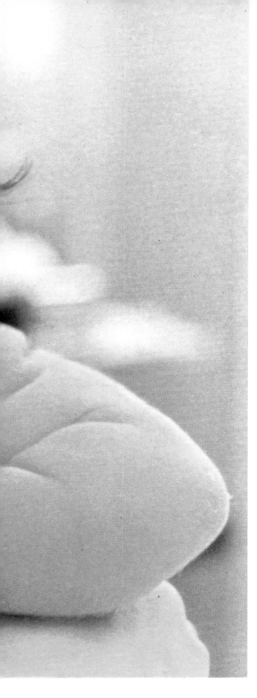

which disappears in a day or so.) The doctor will try to effect a smooth delivery by telling you when to push and not to push. To prevent the sudden expulsion of the baby, he supports the baby's head with his hands.

Most often the baby emerges with his face looking down toward the floor, and then, while his head is held in the doctor's hands, he will turn to one side or the other. Slowly, the doctor will lower the baby's head, easing out the topmost shoulder; then he will raise the head and ease out the other shoulder. The body and legs follow very quickly.

As the head is born, you may see that the umbilical cord is looped around the baby's neck. Don't be alarmed. The doctor will check this immediately. If the cord is loose, he'll slip it over the baby's head; if it's tight, he'll clamp and cut it. If the baby's face is turned the wrong way, forceps may be used to turn his head. If there is a breech presentation and a Caesarian is not necessary, forceps may also to used to help deliver the head.

The mention of forceps causes many women to shudder, and perhaps with good reason if they've heard of difficult forceps deliveries done in the past. But traumatic procedures are seldom attempted any more. If the baby is not well descended, a Caesarian section will be performed. Today, forceps are used to ease the head out gently with less trauma than might occur with prolonged pushing. The blades of the forceps are rounded and smooth and fit the baby's head snugly. They work somewhat like a shoe horn, easing the baby's head past the vaginal opening.

European doctors and some American doctors use a vacuum extractor instead of forceps, which pulls out the baby by means of a suction cup attached to the back of the baby's head. Which is the better instrument has been the subject of some controversy lately. The answer seems to be that the doctor's skill is more important than the particular instrument. In the United States you're more likely to have forceps for the simple reason that your doctor is less likely to have experience with the suction cup. Both instruments work well.

73

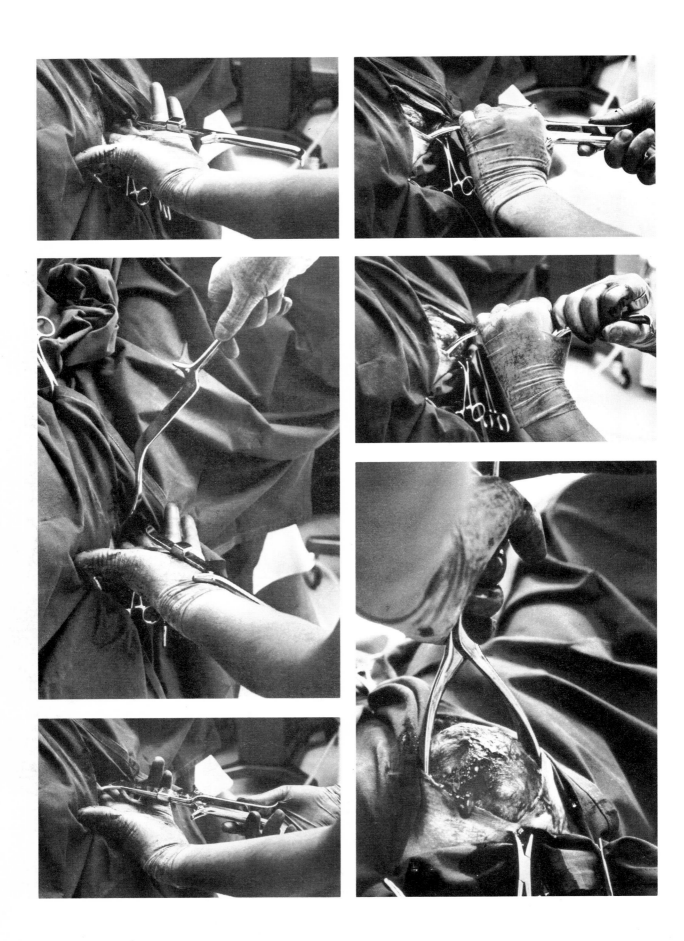

LEFT: *Sometimes forceps are used to minimize the trauma of birth by lifting out a baby who's coming too slowly (or whose mother can't push effectively because of anesthesia).* TOP: *The first forceps' blade (which is not sharp, but rounded and smooth) is introduced and gradually eased into place on one side of the baby's head.* CENTER: *The second blade is guided into the hollow of the sacrum.* BOTTOM: *Then it is turned to the other side of the baby's head.*

NEAR LEFT TOP: *With his left hand, the doctor gives a test tug to be sure the forceps are properly in place and the head is following.* CENTER: *He begins to draw out the baby.* BOTTOM: *A perfect presentation (face downward).*

The head is born. The doctor's right hand guides it past the vaginal opening. The infant is in no way injured. The blood is from the episiotomy and common in a normal birth. If there are any marks at all on the baby, they should clear up in a day or so.

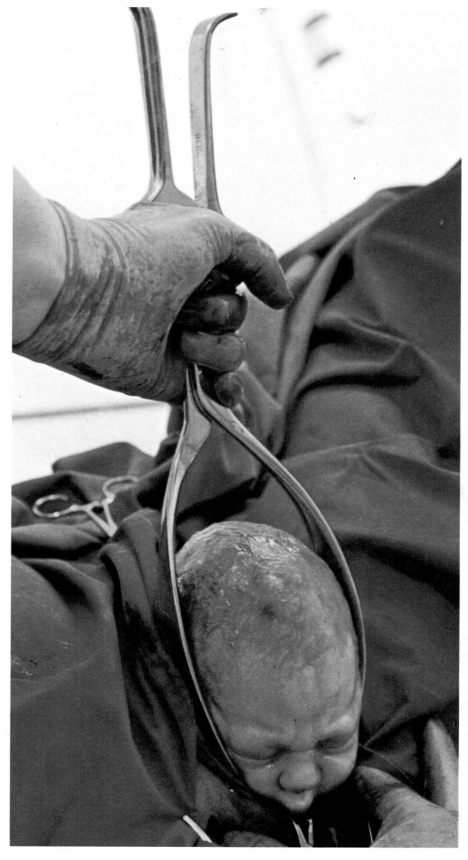

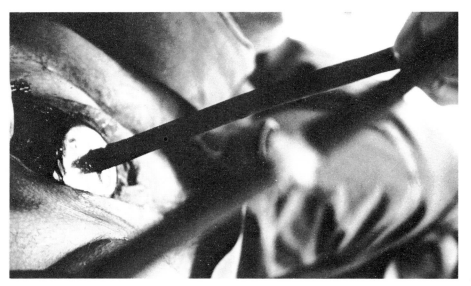

In Europe, many doctors prefer the suction cup to forceps. Here the cup is applied to the baby's head.

And the baby is delivered (along with a gush of amniotic fluid).

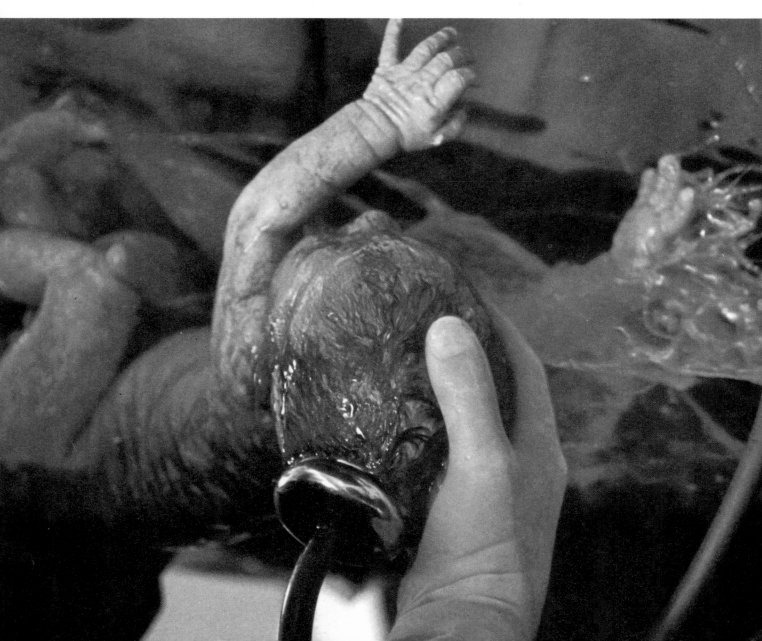

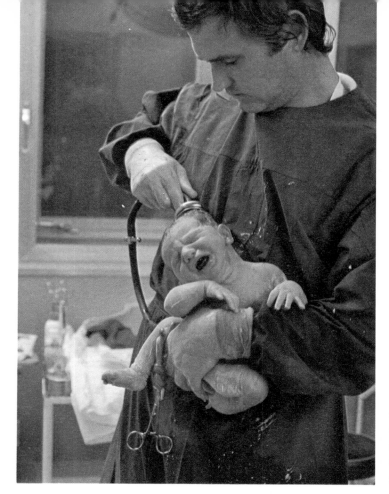

After the baby is breathing and the umbilical cord is clamped, the suction is turned off and the cup is removed.

For a few hours, the mark of the suction cup will be visible on the baby's head. The elongation of the head is primarily the result of normal labor—not the use of suction. It will clear up in a few days.

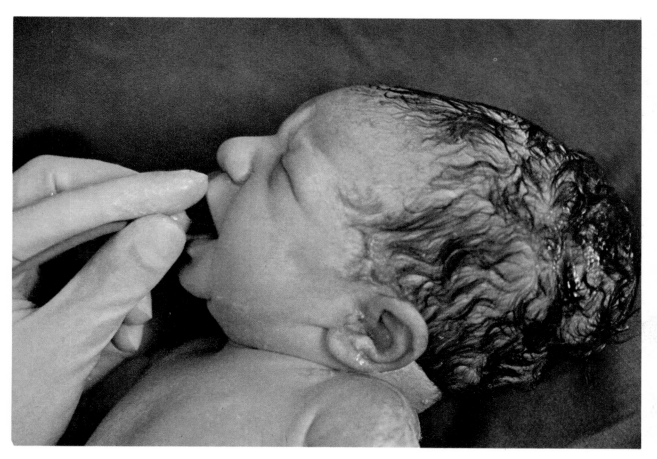

Another focus of controversy is the episiotomy. It is done just before the baby's head is born and when the perineum is greatly distended (so there's ample space for the incision). Some women feel that it's unnecessary in a normal birth and cruel. However, if you're having your first baby or a forceps delivery, your doctor will certainly recommend it. And there are good arguments for it. First, the episiotomy helps to preserve the tone of the perineal muscles, as indicated by the fact that it's associated with fewer problems in later life involving prolapse, or falling, of the uterus and urinary incontinence. Second, it's not considered safe for a first baby to undergo pushing for more than two hours (one hour for a subsequent child); each contraction and depression of the baby's head causes a decrease in heart rate. An episiotomy usually means a quicker delivery (by a half hour to an hour). Finally, an episiotomy prevents tearing of the perineum, which can be difficult to heal.

After delivery of the baby and placenta, the episiotomy will be sewn up. This takes about ten minutes. You may not have any visible stitches or only a few. These don't have to be removed; they'll be absorbed in about a week.

Immediately after delivery, the infant's nose and mouth are sucked free of mucus, and the doctor will keep her in a position with her head down until he's sure the respiratory passages are clear.

Then she has to be wiped dry to prevent her from becoming chilled as the amniotic fluid evaporates from her skin; the head especially must be protected because of its large surface area. There is no reason you cannot nurse immediately if you feel like it, as long as the baby is kept warm. However, your doctor or a nurse or pediatrician also will want to check the baby and you will no doubt sense a certain impatience to get the baby to the nursery. The first assessment of the newborn's status is done in the delivery room, right after birth. The infant is scored on the Apgar scale (devised by Dr. Virginia Apgar) on five criteria: heart rate, respiration, color, muscle tone and reflex irritability. The scale is from zero to ten, and a score of five is considered good. Later, in the nursery, the infant will probably be given a more complete examination by a pediatrician.

It's becoming common to give parents more time with their babies right after birth, and this is certainly welcome. However, the doctors are responsible to be sure that no unforeseen crisis arises in the first moments of the child's life. The baby will soon be all yours.

Recently a great deal of attention has been given to birth techniques advocated by the French physician Frederick Leboyer. He believes that birth as practiced in most hospitals today is an unnecessarily traumatic event for the newborn baby. In his book *Birth Without Violence* he recommends changes to minimize what he feels are the negative aspects of routine institutional procedures. Above all, he asks parents and medical attendants to be more sensitive to the fact that a delicate new life is being born.

Dr. Leboyer suggests a quiet, dimly lit environment and a gentle delivery to soften the impact of the new environment on the baby as he emerges from the womb. If sudden light and abrupt movement are disorienting to all of us, imagine the reaction of a newborn. But Leboyer does believe it is always necessary to have a spotlight on the child as it is being delivered so that its condition can be quickly evaluated. A baby that remains cyanotic (blue, due to low oxygen levels in the blood) or does not breathe immediately upon delivery requires immediate care by the doctor.

At a Leboyer birth, the baby is gently placed on the mother's abdomen immediately after delivery and the umbilical cord is cut only after it has stopped pulsating spontaneously. It is controversial whether delaying the cutting of the cord actually provides any extra oxygen to the baby. After the first breath, pressure changes in the heart automatically close off the valves which allow blood from the cord to flow to the baby's heart. (If the cord is wrapped around the neck of the baby it of course must be clamped before the child can be delivered. This occurs in approximately twenty-five percent of births.)

Dr. Leboyer encourages fathers to be present at birth and to help immediately in the care of their babies. While the baby is on the mother's abdomen, it is gently massaged, preferably by the father. After it is breathing easily, the father (or another attendant at the birth) gives the newborn a warm bath. The idea is that the bath resembles the environment of the womb and provides a familiar sensation to ease the child's adjustment to the world. Also, Dr. Leboyer believes this early contact between the parents and child stimulates bonding—that is, the development of a powerful, mutual intimate relationship between parents and child.

A problem with the Leboyer method is the risk that the infant will become chilled during the massage and bath procedures. As the amniotic fluid evaporates, a newborn's body loses heat rapidly, which can cause serious difficulties. And it isn't easy to maintain a bath at exactly the right temperature. On the other hand, the general approach appeals to common sense, and any safe way to make birth a less difficult experience for the baby is clearly worthwhile. Leboyer's concepts are emotionally stimulating and intellectually interesting.

Dr. Leboyer's methods are being tried in various institutions in the United States. As yet his theories regarding bonding and other supposed benefits of his approach have not been proved scientifically, although he states that the children he has delivered in this fashion are calmer than other children and adjust better to their environment as they grow older. But we do not know whether the expectations of the new parents for a "better child" or the Leboyer method should be given the credit. Undoubtedly at least some of Dr. Leboyer's ideas will become part of the general movement toward making childbirth a more dignified and personally rewarding experience for all—including the child. It is too early to tell whether his specific techniques will find a place in childbirth practices of the future.

Caesarian Birth

Many Caesarian births take place with the mother fully conscious but free of pain and the baby only minimally affected by the drugs used. Apart from the physical advantages of this approach, mother and baby get to meet each other immediately. Too often in the past a Caesarian delivery would cause the mother to feel dissociated from the child—a few hours after birth a drugged and nauseous mother would be presented with a neatly swaddled and also drugged little baby. Not the ideal introduction.

In the days of our great-grandmothers, a Caesarian meant a significant risk to life, and was done only as a last resort, when the mother and/or child was already in trouble. Naturally, as a result, the operation was often done too late. A late-nineteenth-century encyclopedia reads: "A Caesarian section becomes necessary when the foetus is unable to pass through the pelvis, either because the passage is too narrow or the mother has died. In earlier times, the operation on a living patient was extremely dangerous; some half the women undergoing this operation died either immediately because of loss of blood, or later of peritonitis [inflammation of the membrane enveloping most of the viscera]."

Today, we can confidently go ahead with a Caesarian, not only in critical emergencies but to prevent complications while the mother and baby are still strong. And the combination of fetal monitoring and modern surgical techniques has made possible dramatic rescues of babies in trouble. If definite stress is detected in the baby, indicated by a decreased heartbeat or abnormal blood acidity, the mother can rapidly be taken to the operating room, anesthetized and the baby delivered within a few minutes.

Now that Caesarians are apparently so simple and safe, women sometimes think it would be better to have this operation than struggle through a normal delivery. But a Caesarian section is a major abdominal operation and therefore, like any operation, not completely risk-free. It should be avoided whenever possible.

In the recent past there seems to have been something of a fad for

This woman has just been delivered of a daughter by Caesarian section, done with epidural anesthesia. She welcomes her baby while the doctors sew up the wound.

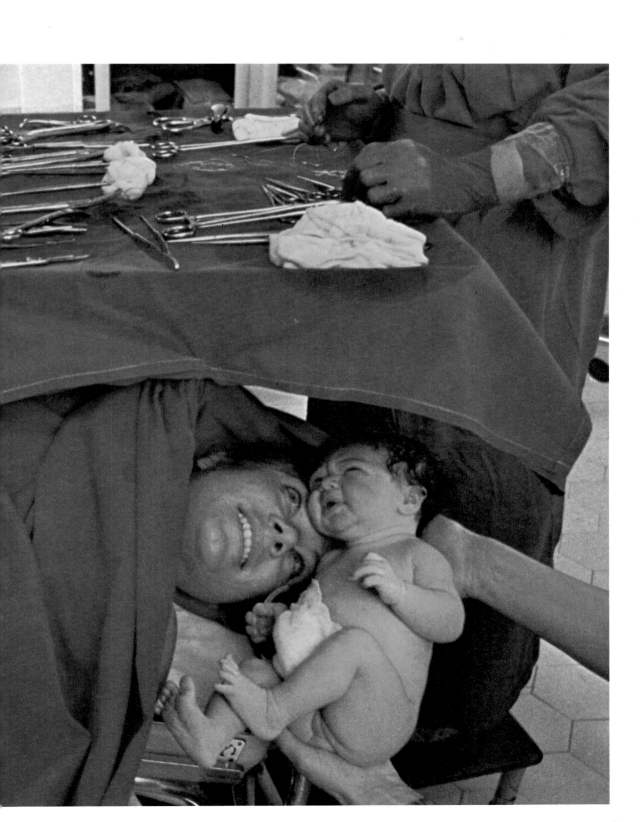

doing Caesarians, and there are still some doctors who do more than are necessary. It may be more convenient to intervene early in a difficult labor with surgery than to wait several hours with an uncomfortable patient to see if a vaginal delivery is possible. However, it's hard to evaluate excessive use of surgery statistically, since the characteristics of the patients involved have to be considered. Caesarians are required quite frequently among women over thirty-five, especially for a first baby, and among girls under sixteen.

The most frequent reason for doing a Caesarian is feto-pelvic disproportion; in other words, the baby is too big to pass through the woman's pelvis. It's difficult to diagnose this condition before labor begins, but if your doctor suspects it exists, he may order pelvic X-rays in your last month of pregnancy or during early labor. And even with the X-rays, he still may not be certain what will happen. In most cases, the best way to evaluate the situation is to allow the woman to go into labor and observe the baby's progress carefully.

If your doctor decides you should have a Caesarian, this isn't usually an acute emergency, and you may be asked whether you prefer an epidural anesthetic, which will leave you conscious while the baby's born, or a general anesthetic. It's a good idea to talk over with your doctor ahead of time under what circumstances he would consider a Caesarian and any questions you have about the possible anesthetics.

Before the operation with an epidural, you maybe given a tranquilizer to calm any nervousness. After the baby is delivered, you may then be given a light dose of a general anesthetic, such as nitrous oxide.

A Caesarian generally takes about an hour, with the baby being delivered in the first five minutes and the rest of the time spent on repairing the wounds. For cosmetic reasons, a low, horizontal incision just above the pubic bone is preferred; the scar will be hidden by the pubic hair. But a longitudinal incision down the middle of the abdomen may be indicated for a woman with extremely narrow hips having a large baby.

How quickly a mother wakes up after a Caesarian and regains her strength depends on a number of factors. If she's been through a long and tiring labor prior to the operation she may awaken only briefly and then sleep for many hours. If she's gone into the operation fresh, she may be alert after a couple of hours, able to hold and even breast feed her baby.

The amount of discomfort experienced following the surgery is extremely variable. But no matter how much pain you feel, the best cure is to start moving around as soon as possible. The nurses aren't trying to torture you when they insist you get up and take a few steps. Activity promotes the restoration of normal respiration, digestion and excretion. Inactivity can lead to respiratory infection and gas pains—which can be worse than your original pains, especially since you don't get as much sympathy.

Caesarian babies are usually very pretty, not having been battered about in a vaginal birth like most of their neighbors in the nursery. In fact, you might wonder why nature hasn't arranged for all babies to pop out effortlessly. Aside from the necessity of guarding against accidental expulsion of the baby, nature's method also serves to stimulate the baby's major physiological systems by the pressure of the contractions. Among many animals it seems that not only is the natural labor important to the offspring, but that the licking the mother gives her babies after birth is a continuation of the labor process and helps the little creatures off to a good start in breathing, eating and digesting. Among humans, Caesarian babies are watched extra closely at first to be sure they're breathing properly.

Otherwise, Caesarian babies are as healthy as any others, and there are mothers who swear they're more easygoing babies. It's true that a Caesarian baby comes into the world with less physical trauma than a baby who's been through a long and rigorous labor. So perhaps they do tend to be more relaxed.

After a Caesarian delivery, your doctor will probably want you to remain in the hospital for about a week, mostly to be sure that no complications develop, such as fever or poor healing of the wound. But you can breast feed your baby and do just about everything you could have done with a normal delivery. When you return home, it may take longer than you expect to recover your strength, so be careful not to rush into a full schedule.

You will be able to have more children if you want, unless there was some unusual complication. Your doctor will probably, but not necessarily, recommend that your next child be delivered by Caesarian. If you'd like to try a vaginal delivery, discuss this with him.

If you're scheduled for a Caesarian and know that you don't want any more children, you can ask your doctor to do a tubal ligation during the operation. This permanent method of sterilization entails cutting the Fallopian tubes so that the eggs produced by the ovaries cannot be reached by sperm. Many women find this the ideal method of birth control, involving little risk, no effort and almost no possibility of failure. Your hormonal cycle will continue as before and you'll continue to ovulate and menstruate.

The question that's asked more than any other about modern Caesarians is, "What does it feel like?" Many women have such a queasy feeling about the procedure that they reject epidural anesthesia and ask to be put under completely, which is perfectly legitimate to do. If you think you might have panicky reactions, you should say so. An anxious patient with soaring blood pressure is at unnecessary risk. On the other hand, some women want to be wide awake and object even to a routine tranquilizer.

The following quotes from women who've delivered with an epidural anesthetic are characteristic reactions to the experience:

The mother lies on her side and her back is painted with a disinfectant. Then the injection is given.

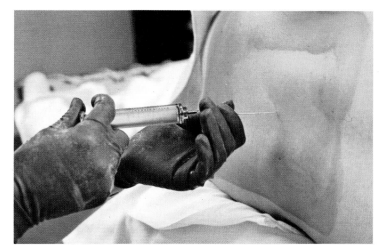

The anesthetic begins to take effect immediately.

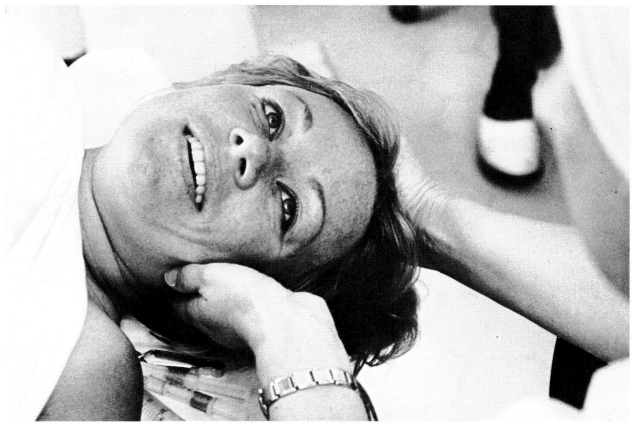

"Epidural anesthesia was something quite new for me, of course. I was a bit excited. When I lay down on my side on the operating table, I thought to myself, I hope the shot doesn't hurt. Someone painted the disinfection stuff on a large part of my back. The fluid quickly evaporated. It smelled like iodine. The syringe was like one used for an ordinary injection, only a little longer. I had to relax totally and not move at all. The needle stung a bit. Instantly, I had no more sensation down below. They turned me over on my back again. The blue cloths were spread over me. At the same time, my arms and legs were strapped down. The instrument table emerged into my limited field of vision. And now I waited, curious but not anxious, for the operation to begin. Lying in that small cave, I felt glad that the anesthetist was present. She explained what was happening with my body. The three surgeons didn't say a word. Only the instruments clacked lightly. 'Now the abdominal wall is open. Did it hurt?' No, I hadn't felt anything of the long cut, except for a remote sense of contact."

"Retrospectively, I think that the doctors underestimated me a little. Naturally, they only wanted the best thing for me. I wasn't to have any anxieties whatsoever. Some women probably have a vestigial doubt about whether the anesthesia will really block pain one hundred percent. Total anesthesia is pretty clear because you're unconscious. Only a few hospitals have epidural anesthesia. And since very few women have their Caesarian by this method, there's a lack of experience. It hasn't really gotten around what a fantastic thing this is: You're cut open, you remain fully conscious and you don't feel the least pain. It's really sensational. It sounds incredible. Even I couldn't believe it until the very last instant. At any rate, the doctors were smart enough to give me a tranquilizer in advance. It was pretty strong. I was *slightly high, and for moments at a time I felt sleepy. I must have actually slept for about five minutes. My sense of time got all muddled during the operation. At times, everything seemed to be going very fast, at times very slowly. Retrospectively, I'm sorry they gave me a tranquilizer. After all, the doctors couldn't know how curious I was about the birth. But my anesthetist had her reasons for her decision. According to the old operating-room rule, the anesthetist is the pilot and the surgeon the captain."*

"If the anesthetist hadn't said to me: 'Now we're starting,' I wouldn't have noticed. Unfortunately, the doctor had to concentrate so heavily on her work that she couldn't explain what was happening. Everything was so discreet, so calm. I would have much preferred watching. I know that a Caesarian can be a bloody operation, but I'm not afraid of blood, not even my own. It would have been very important for me to see my own flesh and blood, my child, from the very beginning. Instead, I merely lay in the stillness and waited for the first cry. For a long time nothing happened. Then my whole body was slightly shaken. The slight shakes came periodically, several times. Now I realized: They're drawing my child out of my abdomen. There were supposedly only seven minutes between the first cut and the first cry. But it seemed much longer. And then the cry I had been longing for. Everything had gone well. Thank goodness! I wanted to see my child immediately, I tried to sit up, but I couldn't. I was strapped down, after all. Oh, how blissful I was, hearing that cry. It wasn't a cry of happiness. It was more like a protest. I had not seen the child yet, and I thought to myself: 'I hope they put a few warm things on him, he must be freezing.' Then they showed me a coppery, beautiful child. Completely different from what I had imagined. Beautiful, but alien. I was absolutely flabbergasted."

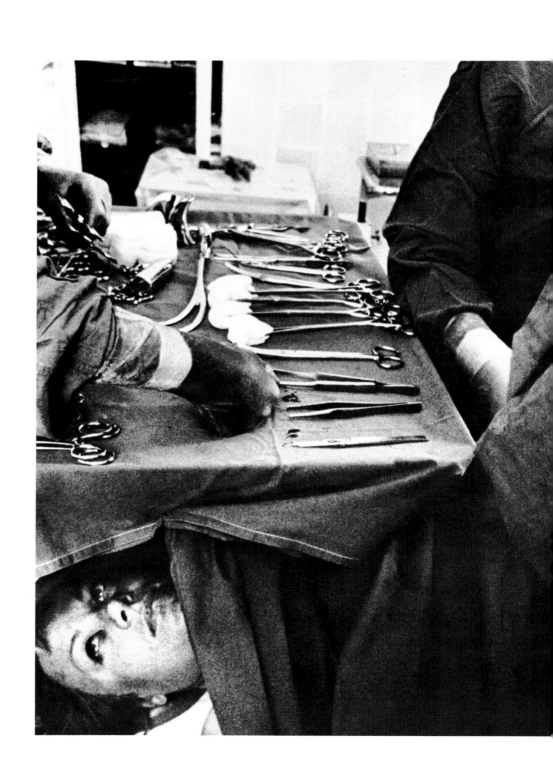

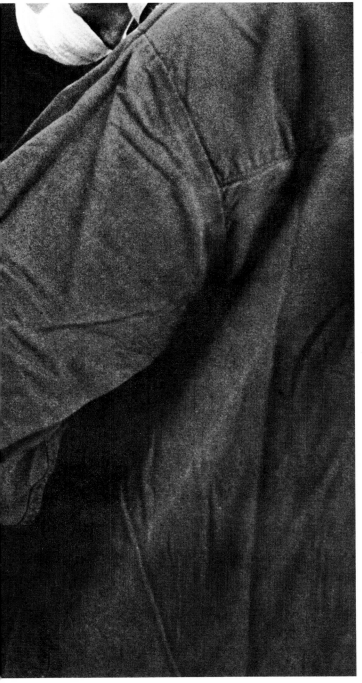

The mother is concerned, but doesn't feel the incision. (In the United States, the instrument table is kept over the woman's feet.)

The face emerges first. A suction cup or one blade of the forceps may be used to lift up the head. The bluish lips are normal. The child is calm and seems to be asleep.

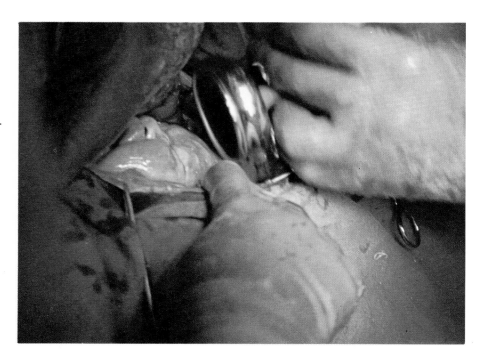

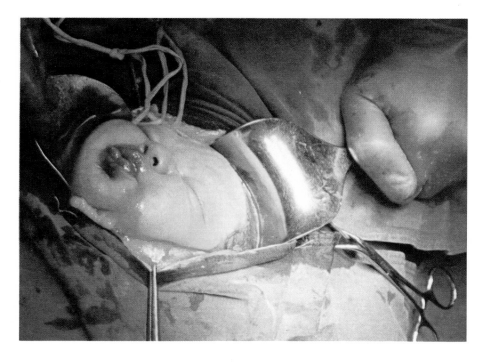

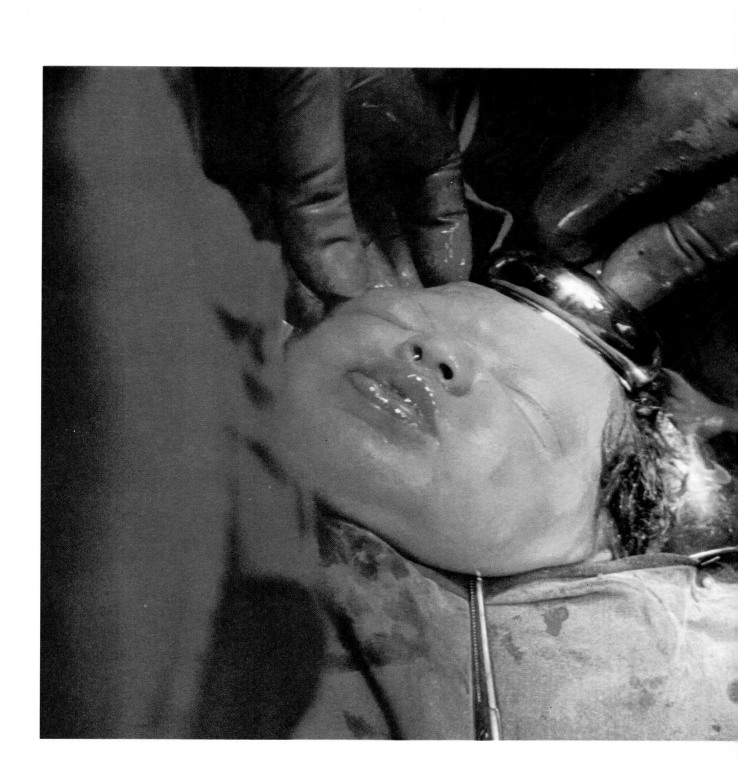

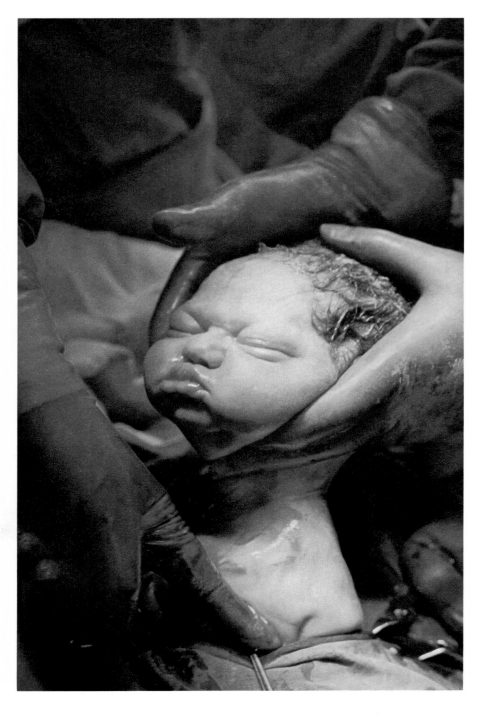

And presented immediately to her mother.

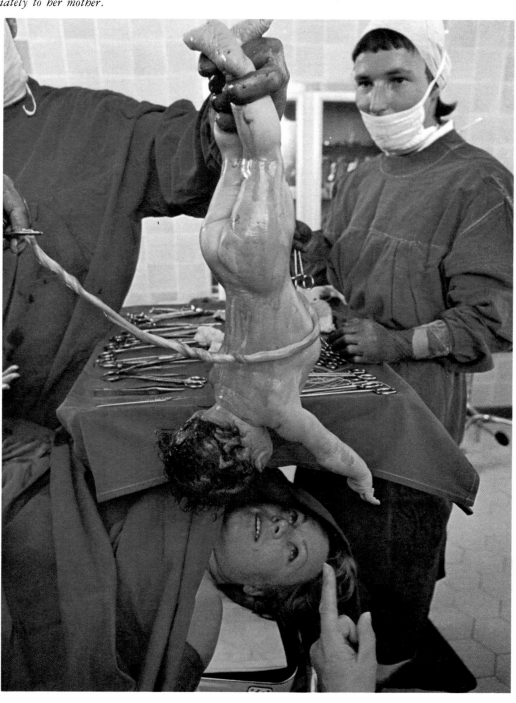

"The feeling: Now it's here. They put the child right next to my face. I didn't care whether it was a boy or a girl. My husband had wanted a girl. And it was a girl. The main thing for me was: It's healthy, it's all right, the child's doing fine. Other women say they were overcome with a maternal feeling from the very first instant. Curiosity, amazement, relief and a bit of pride—those were my first sensations. I wanted to get to know this strange person. I did know that this was our little daughter. Although I saw, smelled and felt her up close, she still seemed strange. But I did know that I would soon love my child."

Feeling the touch of her mother, the little girl's fingers grasp for her.

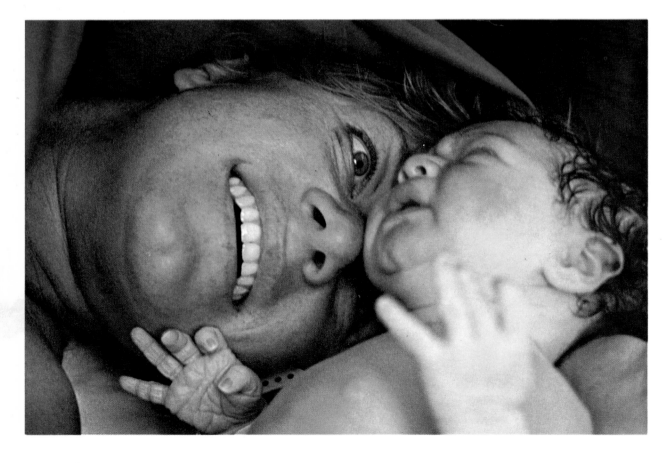

Twins

Twins are special. The womb is designed to carry one baby. When there are two, the space is tight and the mother's physiological resources are strained. As a result, twins are usually born a few weeks early and are usually small for their age. But compared with a single baby of the same weight, say 5½ pounds, a small twin is hardier because his total development is more advanced.

Twins are sometimes a surprise. You may not know you've been blessed until after one child is born and your doctor announces, "There's another one in there!" You won't be the only person in the delivery room who's excited. Twin births are a challenge that keeps everyone busy, and this is an appropriate introduction to becoming the mother of twins. You can expect to be kept busy for quite a few years.

The chances are about seventy percent that your doctor or midwife will detect twins before labor starts. The most obvious sign is that the uterus is larger than normal; this is most apt to be detected near the end of the second trimester. A sure diagnosis, however, is a little tricky. The doctor will attempt to distinguish two heartbeats, but sometimes one interferes with another. Sonography should provide a definite diagnosis, but there have been cases in which sonographs haven't revealed the second baby, because one twin was lying on top of the other. Of course, it is often the woman herself who mentions the possibility of twins. A woman who's had one or more children already can often tell the difference when she's carrying twins. Unusually lively fetal motion is one sign.

You're more likely to have twins 1) as you get older; 2) if you've already had one or more children, and 3) if there are twins in your family or the father's. Fraternal twins, which develop from two separate eggs fertilized by separate sperm, are far more common than identical twins, which develop from one egg and one sperm. The latter are genetically identical, whereas fraternal twins can be different sexes, and even when they're the same sex, their appearance may be very different. Identical twins can be almost impossible to tell apart,

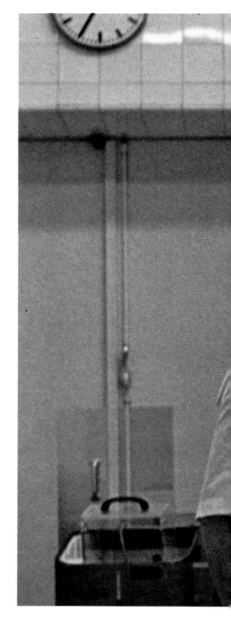

When twins are expected, extra people are at hand to help.

and the parents have to take care to help each one develop his or her own sense of individuality. In cases in which it isn't clear whether twins are fraternal or identical, genetic testing can provide the answer.

The woman pregnant with twins generally has a more difficult time of it. She's more prone to develop toxemia; toward the end of pregnancy, she may simply feel overburdened, with good reason, and there's a greater possibility of a premature labor. If you're carrying twins, it's important to see your doctor regularly and to rest. If early changes in your cervix indicate that a premature delivery is possible,

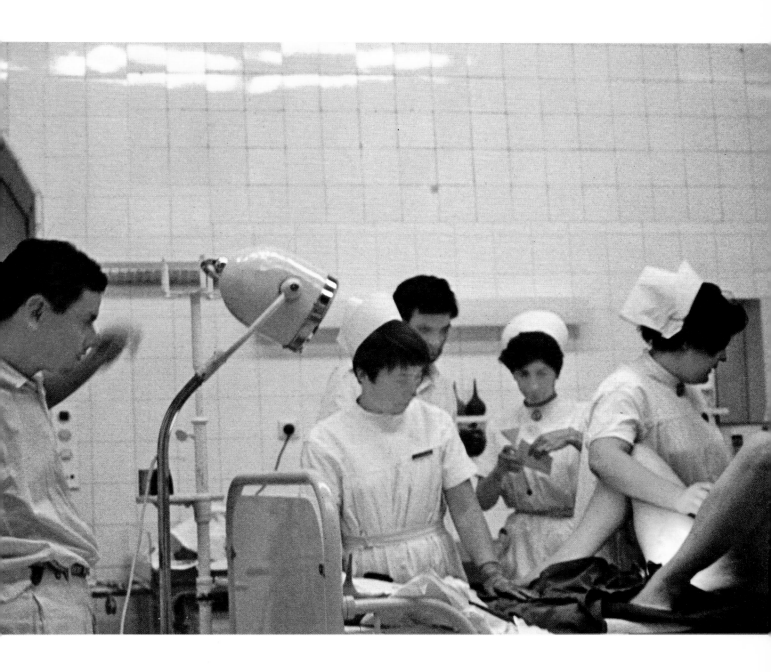

your doctor may tell you to stay in bed. The longer the delivery is postponed, the better.

Labor with twins is often shorter and easier than usual, but may not be forceful enough to push out the babies, especially the second one. After the first baby is born, the doctor ordinarily waits a few minutes to see if the second will come spontaneously. If this doesn't happen in five to fifteen minutes, the doctor will intervene. He'll rupture the second amniotic sac, if it's intact, and lift out the baby, with the help of forceps or suction if necessary.

Often in the case of twins one baby is a breech presentation or is

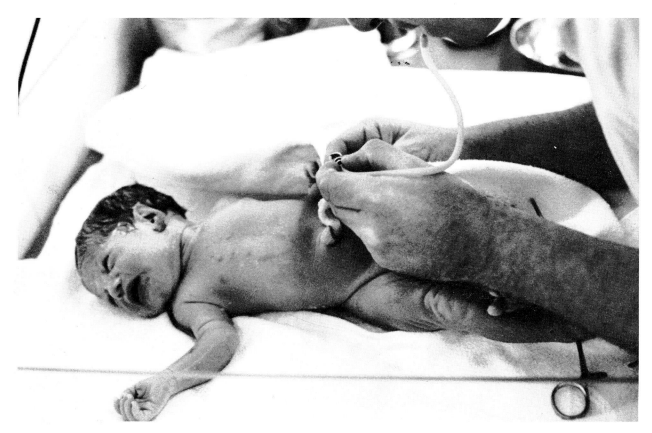

lying in a transverse position, i.e., sideways. This may complicate the delivery to the point that a Caesarian has to be done.

Twins have a special place in parents' hearts, perhaps because of the effort that goes into raising them. If you have twins unexpectedly, reevaluate the plans you've made for the near future. Many women are dismayed by the amount of work needed to care for one baby—twins require twice the work. Whatever help you can get, from friends, relatives or employees, take it. And the father should be prepared to share in the mothering; he's going to be needed.

If you'd planned to breast feed, you still can with twins. You may

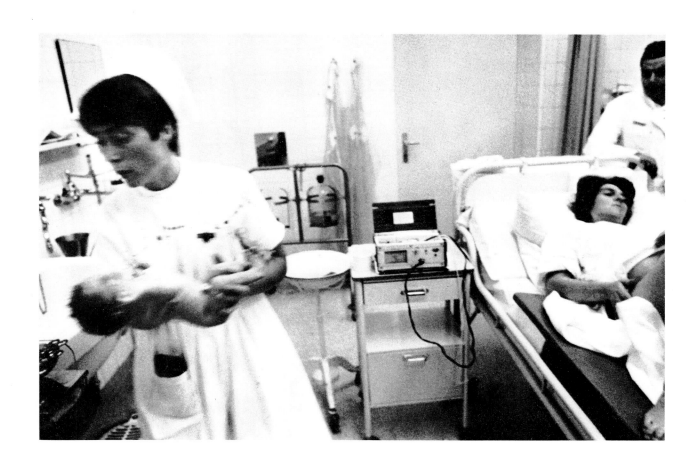

have to go over to the bottle after a while, but whatever time they get at the breast is good for them, and probably more convenient for you. Preparing formula, sterilizing bottles and so on for two is a lot of trouble.

As your children grow, you'll find that everyone has some theory or other on how to raise twins, and no matter what you do, you're going to be told it's wrong. If your children are generally happy, don't worry about it. Twins have some special difficulties (for example, they have to learn to share their parents' attention) and some special advantages (such as companionship). Like any child, a twin

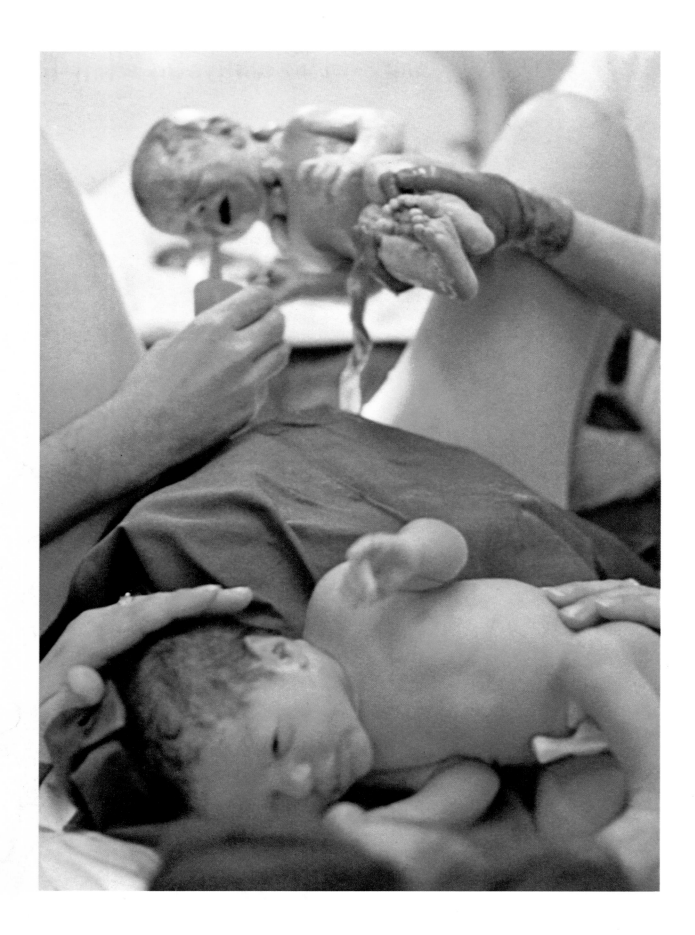

Mother and daughter greet each other while doctors attend to her son.

The baby girl is having a plastic clamp attached to the cut end of the umbilical cord. A blood sample is being taken from the boy.

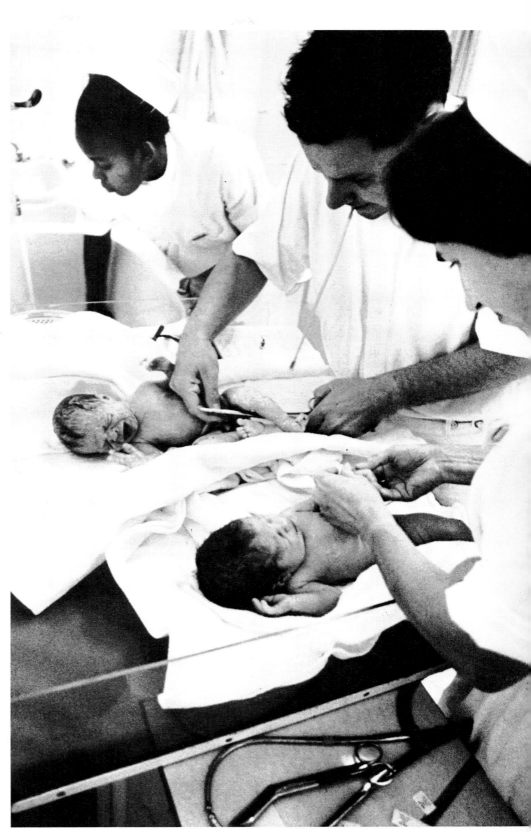

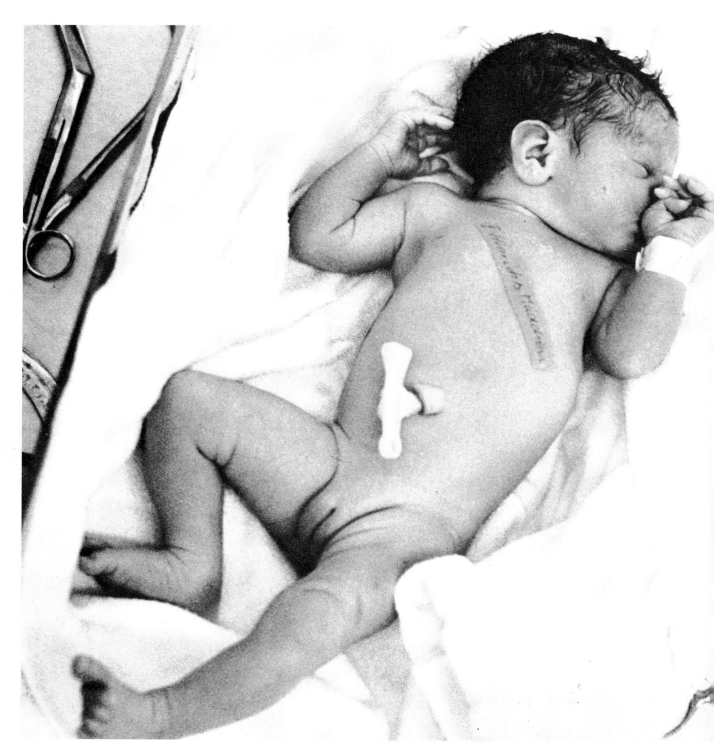

The sister, only ten minutes older, already seems at home in the world.

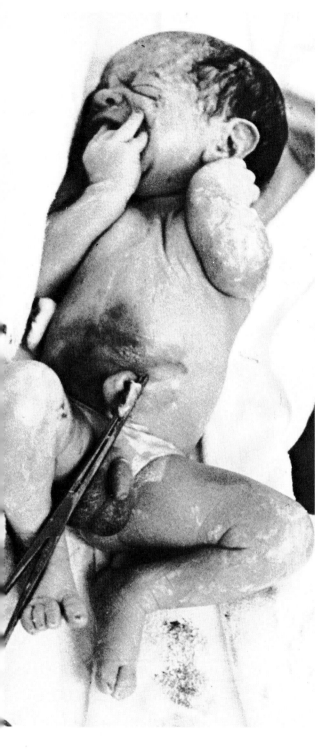
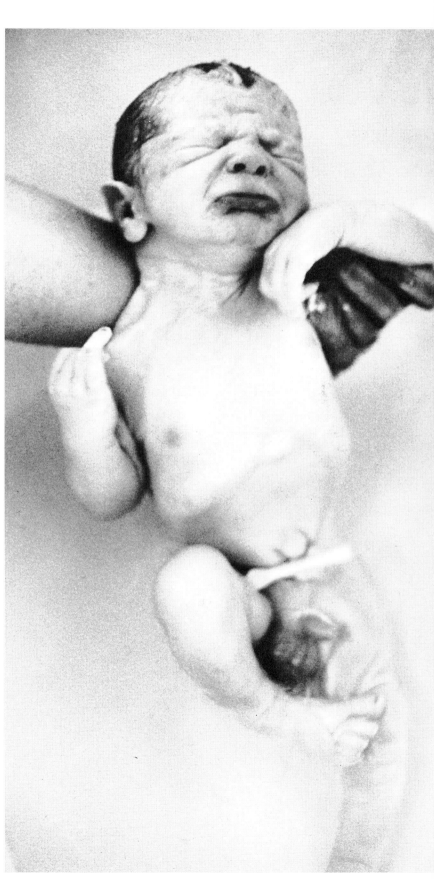

His first bath. Despite his expression, the water is warm. (In the United States, babies are usually just wiped down.)

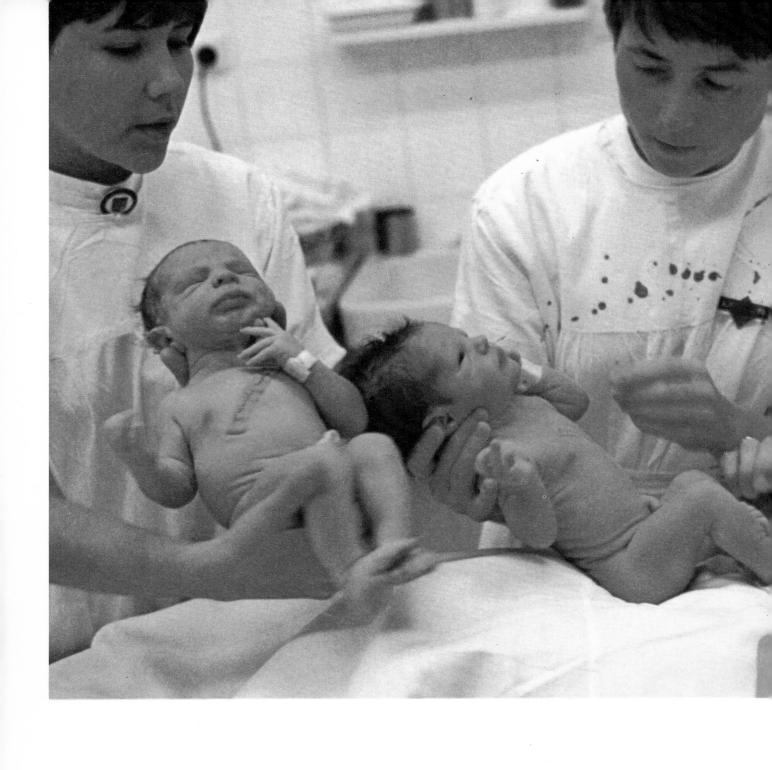

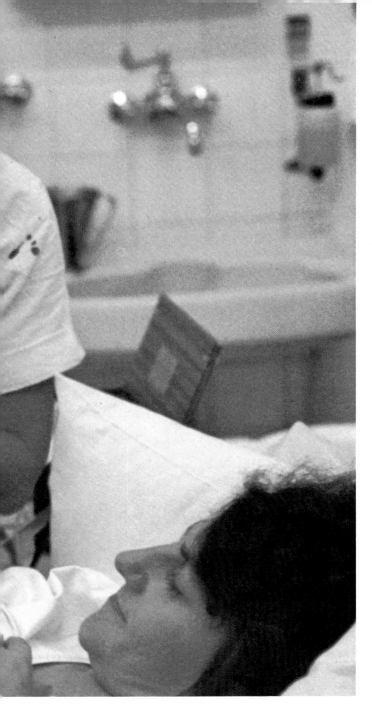

Both are finally ready for their mother's inspection.

will let you know what he or she wants and needs if you're listening.

The raising of twins is simple compared to raising three or more babies, but such multiple births are becoming more and more common due to the use of several so-called "fertility drugs" that stimulate ovulation. These substances fairly often cause the release of more than one ovum at a time, and two or more may be fertilized almost simultaneously. If you're being treated with such a drug, both you and the father should be prepared psychologically for this possibility, and realize that with three or more infants, some or all of them may fail to survive. Luckily, the parents who undertake fertility treatments are usually stoic about the risks and delighted with the baby or babies they bring into the world.

Premature Birth

Today, many seven- and most eight-month babies have a good chance for survival, and even some younger ones as well. Medically, a baby is considered premature if it weighs between 2 pounds, 4 ounces (1,000 grams) and 5½ pounds (2,500 grams). The survival rate varies from twenty percent to over ninety percent, depending on a variety of factors. The majority of the tiniest infants do not live, but the majority of infants 3½ to 4½ pounds do survive with special care. A premature newborn is immediately put into intensive care. The first several days are the most critical period. The longer a child lives, the greater are his chances for survival.

It's important to know exactly how premature the baby is. Prematurity is related to the true age of the infant. This is determined not only by his weight and measurements but also by the physical and laboratory findings that tell the doctors how mature (developed) the infant is. Among the physical findings, weight, length, size of the head, development of the nipples, genitals and earlobes are evaluated. Neurological age is determined by a number of responses, including the infant's ability to grasp and body movement when shaken suddenly.

When a baby comes into the world ahead of time, he needs an environment that resembles the uterus, which is what an incubator is designed to provide. Prototypes of the modern design were first introduced in the early thirties, and there have been numerous improvements since then. The most immediate need of a premature baby is for warmth and dampness. The immature organism can't yet properly control its body temperature, since the smaller the body, the greater the relative surface area of skin; heat is lost at a critically rapid rate. The temperature in an incubator is kept about 95°F. The humidity is kept at seventy to ninety percent to prevent the paper-thin skin and the mucous membranes of the respiratory tract from drying out.

Breathing is a strain for premature babies. They often have periods when they do not breathe effectively. To detect this, sensitive electrodes are attached to the chest to register the heartbeat and breathing rhythm. The younger the child, the greater the danger of hyaline membrane disease. This is a type of respiratory distress due to pulmonary immaturity, but contemporary medical care has also improved the chances of infants affected with this disease.

If the infant's blood is low in oxygen, this can be supplied directly into the incubator. Oxygen levels are carefully monitored. This is because too much oxygen can also be harmful to the infant, resulting in a form of blindness called retrolental fibroplasia and even in breathing problems.

A premature child, even a relatively strong one, has an appearance very different from a full-term baby's. She's all skin and bones (and relatively soft bones, at that). She has no baby fat or chubby, delightful curves. Even if she is able to feed, there's a danger that her breathing and sucking mechanisms may become confused, causing choking. The doctor may prescribed a fluid diet to be administered directly into the baby's blood system. Usually, this is done by inserting an I.V. into a vein. Sometimes, it is put in a vein under the skin of the baby's head, because the veins are easy to find here and the newborn cannot reach the area with her hands and dislodge it.

All infants have incomplete liver function at birth. This is significant because the liver helps to clear bilirubin (a yellow pigment) from the blood. Premature infants have more difficulty with this problem. The liver can become overworked and an increasing jaundice (yellow color) may develop. At signs of increasing jaundice, a special fluorescent light may be turned on over the incubator. This light helps break down the bilirubin. If such phototherapy isn't adequate, the physician may try a blood exchange.

Sophisticated care of the premature requires an enormous expenditure of technical, financial and especially human resources. But it is well worth it when lives are saved.

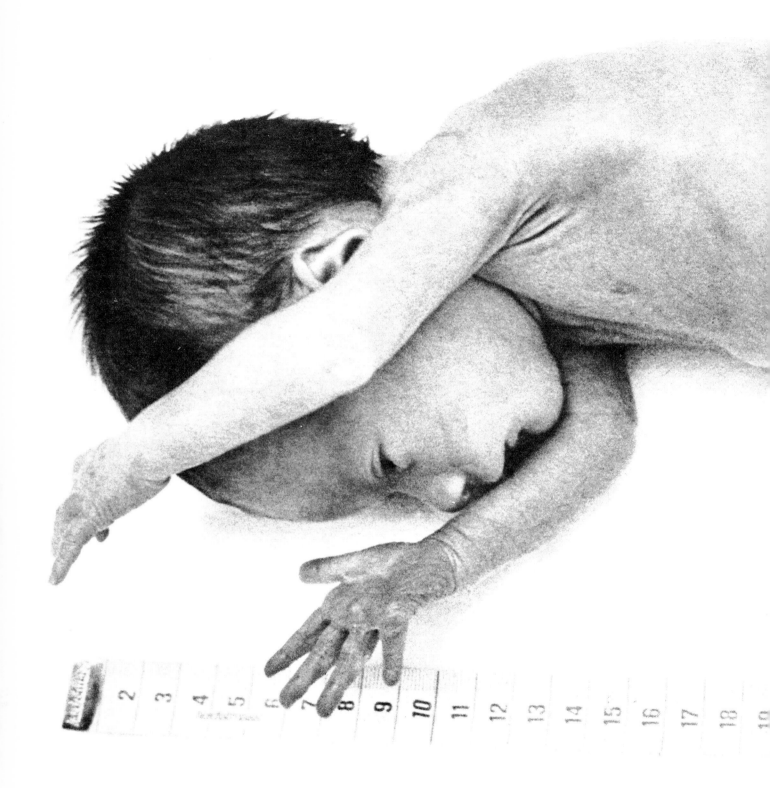

This baby (shown life-size) was born five weeks early. He is now twenty-one days old and weighs over three pounds. Thanks to the modern incubator, his prospects for survival and a normal life are excellent.

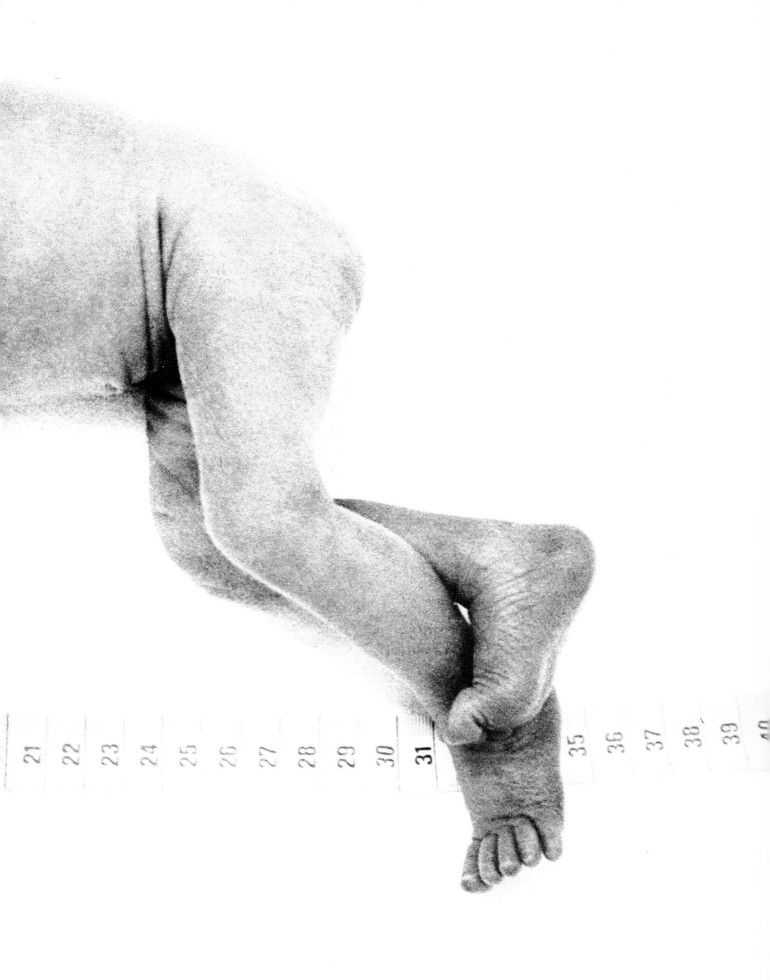

21 22 23 24 25 26 27 28 29 30 **31** 35 36 37 38 39

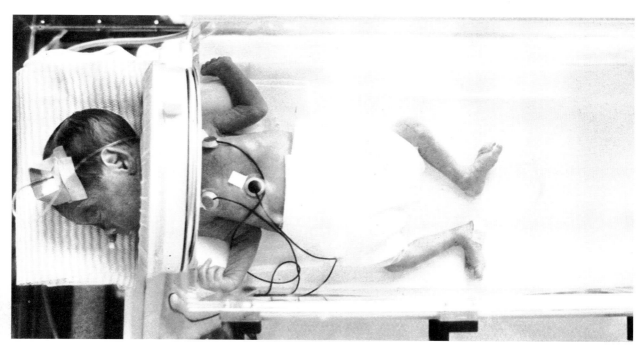

A premature infant in a low-pressure chamber that allows the lungs to expand more easily. Electrodes monitor the heartbeat and respiration. An I.V. on top of the head supplies nourishment.

The child's head rests on sterile cloths. A nasal tube is kept in place in case oxygen is needed.

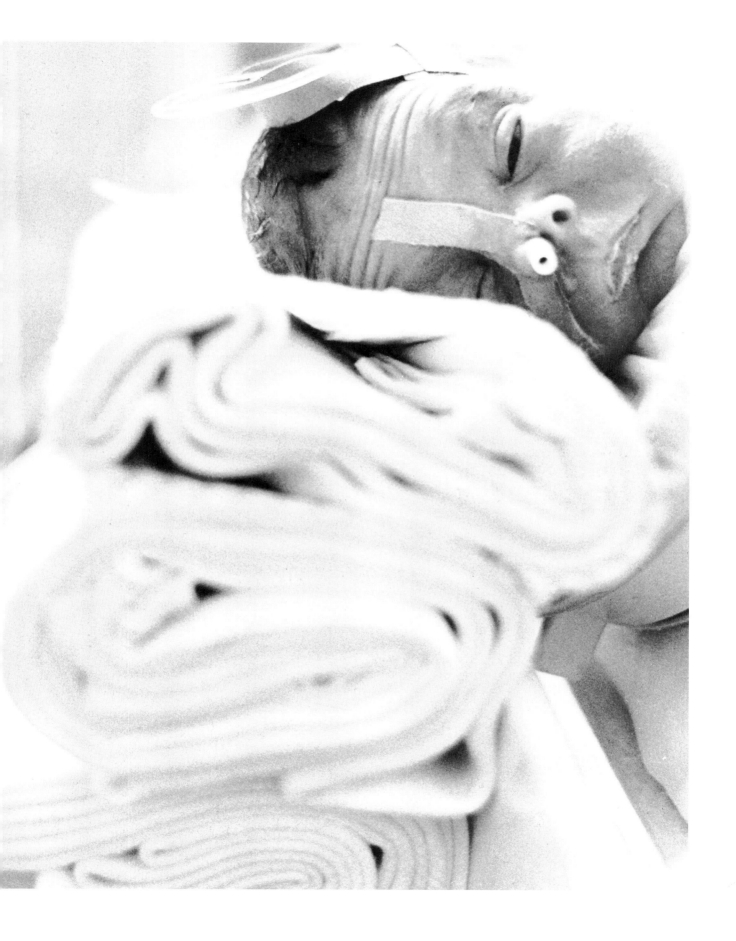

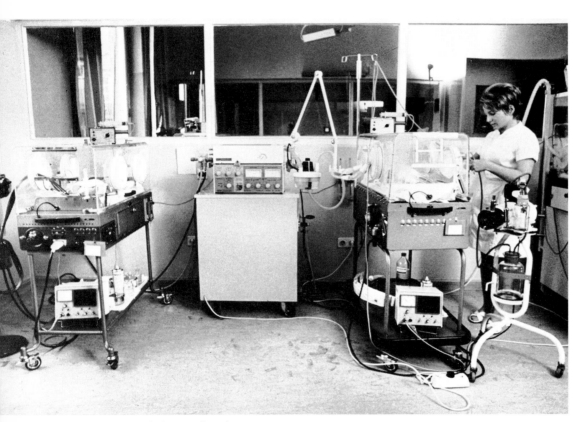
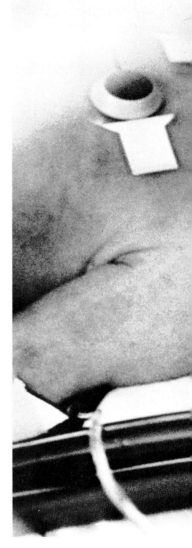

A premature baby ward with
incubators, pumps, monitors
and I.V. equipment (Pediatric
Hospital, University of Munich).

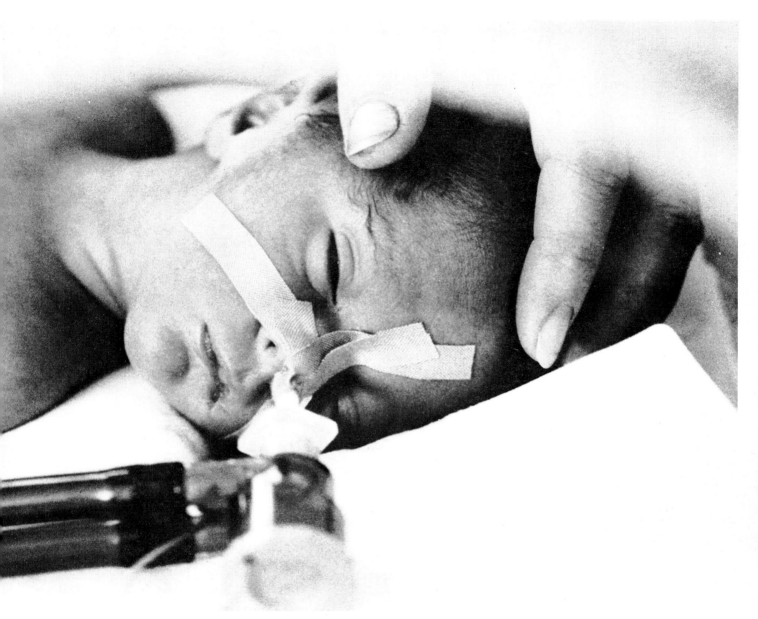

*A weak sleepy infant is given
oxygen and comforted by the
touch of a hand.*

At birth a premature baby differs in many ways from a full-term one. The feet (see right) are smooth, almost unlined. At term, the feet are wrinkled and strongly lined. A premature's hands are frail and can't grasp. The outer ears are still soft and can be folded easily. Later, the cartilage will develop.

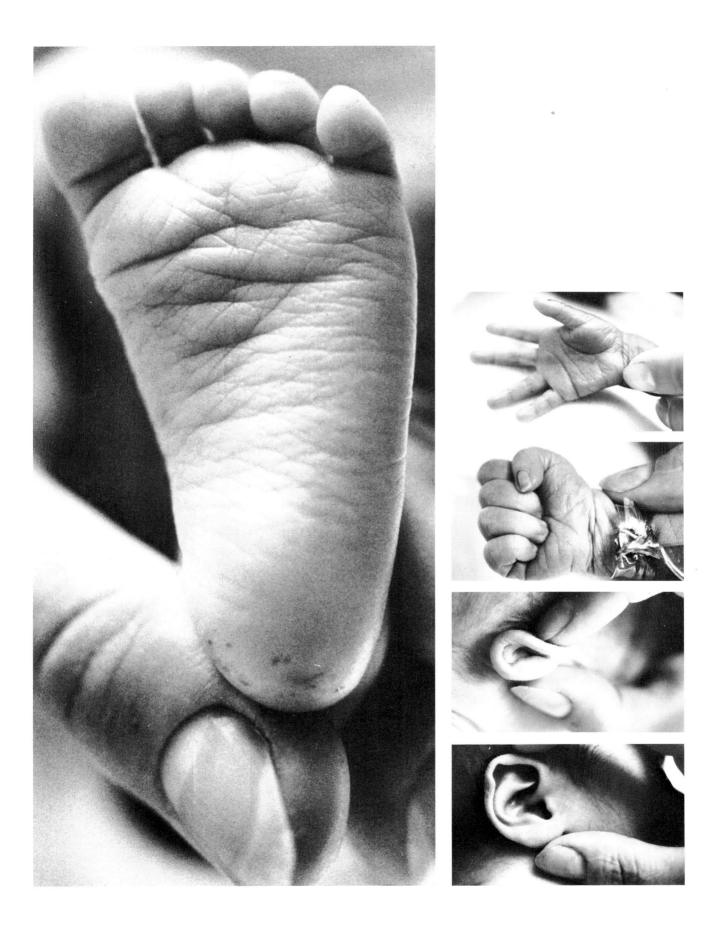

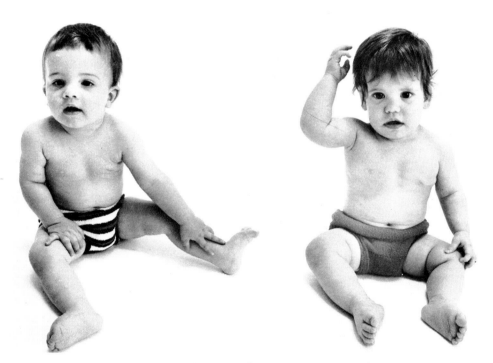

Premature babies catch up quickly. Which of these two boys was a seven-month baby? The one on the right. A year ago he weighed only half as much as his neighbor in the striped pants.

Midwives

Midwives have been referred to often in this book, but in the United States many women have never met a midwife, and have no idea what kind of care they're trained to give. Recently, there's been considerable publicity about the benefits of being cared for by a midwife, but in many parts of the country it still may be difficult to locate one. Much of the interest in midwifery has arisen among women searching for new approaches to childbirth and their concern about the relationship between themselves and the individual providing maternity care.

Historically, the profession of nurse-midwifery was first recognized in the United States in 1925, when the Frontier Nursing Service began a demonstration project in the backhills of Kentucky under the direction of Mary Breckenridge, who along with the nurse-midwives she supervised had been trained in Great Britain. There and in West European countries such as the Netherlands and West Germany, the majority of maternity patients traditionally have been cared for by nurse-midwives. These countries also have among the lowest infant mortality and morbidity rates (the United States ranks seventeenth in infant mortality). One reason may be that midwives are educated to trust and respect natural processes and to interfere as little as possible with the natural forces of birth.

The term "midwife" still conjures up a vision of a "granny" without formal medical training. But the modern American nurse-midwife is a highly educated and trained professional. The Maternity Center Association in New York City established the first American school of midwifery in 1931. (And in 1976 they established the Childbearing Center, where prenatal care and births are conducted by nurse-midwives with the supervision of a staff of M.D.'s; an alternative to hospital-based care, the Center meets rigid state and city health-code standards.) The training was patterned on the English system, and students were drawn from among practicing public-health nurses. At present, there are approximately 2,100 nurse-midwives certified by the American College of Nurse-Midwives (ACNM), and about half of

Checking the baby's heartbeat with a fetoscope.

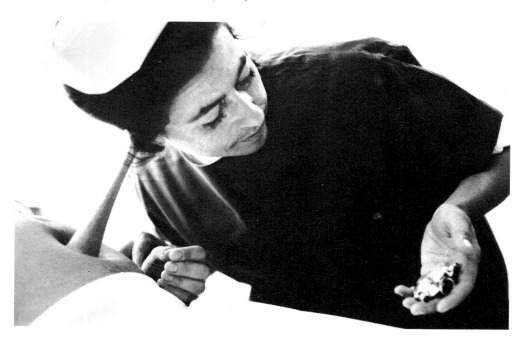

these women are actively practicing midwifery. There are also about 250 midwifery students in seventeen schools across the country.

A midwife is trained first in general nursing and then in her specialization. Her education covers the knowledge necessary to manage a normal pregnancy, labor and delivery, and to recognize variances from the norm. But in midwifery, as opposed to medical training, the emotional and social aspects of the maternity cycle are also emphasized. The certified nurse-midwife is entitled to use the initials CNM after her signature and is eligible to apply to practice midwifery.

Many couples from many different backgrounds have found CNMs more sympathetic and helpful than obstetricians during pregnancy. One reason is undoubtedly that the midwife sees her role as one of helping a couple through all aspects of pregnancy. She is able to give guidance in general health, explain and manage labor and delivery, answer questions about care of the mother and baby after birth and offer psychological support. A doctor is trained with far more emphasis on the treatment of disease than on preventive approaches or teaching techniques. If there's nothing wrong with a patient, he may feel there's nothing for him to do.

Nurse-midwifery is sometimes considered primarily a means of providing inexpensive health care to the poor. But this is a narrow view of a potentially far more valuable profession and, in fact, it is well-to-do and educated women who have sought out midwives and publicized their work. These women have rejected the depersonalizing aspects of routine obstetrical care, and have demanded a more relaxed, concerned and intimate relationship. In particular, many value having a woman to turn to.

Some pregnant women who are alienated from the medical establishment turn to home delivery with midwifery care. But very few CNMs do home deliveries. The CNM tends to see herself as an innovator within the system, promoting new ways for women to have children with greater dignity, comfort and safety. Midwives have been among the first to try new positions for labor and delivery, early-labor lounges and managing labor and birth in the same room. At the same time, most midwives want to have available sophisticated resources for any woman or baby in trouble.

A CNM and doctor consult and work together and complement each other. Most American midwives are full-time hospital staff members. But increasing numbers are joining in independent practice with a doctor or group of doctors. As the profession of midwifery grows, more pregnant women will have a more extensive and less expensive type of care within their reach.

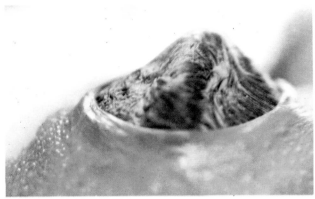

A midwife and nurse encourage a mother with her pushing. The head is coming!

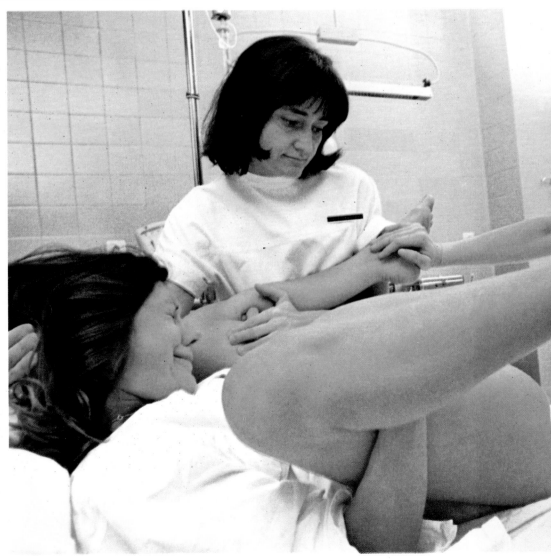

Lying-In

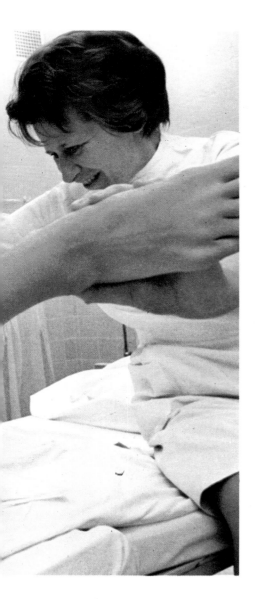

"You're here. You're healthy. You're beautiful. You're my baby. I carried you under my heart for nine months. I was the shell, you were the pearl. Now I hold you in my arms, my delicate jewel. You're tender and precious. Your skin is so soft, your body so fine. My eyes can't get enough of you. I have to touch you, caress you. I cover you with kisses. You smell so sweet. I'm amazed that such a darling creature was born from me. I'm always with you. Don't cry, little baby. I'll feed you. You won't lack a thing. I'll wash you, I'll keep you warm. I'll watch over you when you sleep. When you're cheerful, so am I. You're still weak: I'll protect you. You're still small: You'll grow. You need me. I need you. I'm your mother, and you're my child. Today our life together begins."

Many new mothers, like this one, are filled with joy. Others ache and are depressed, don't know how to relate to their babies and feel isolated. Many fluctuate between happiness and misery.

It will help if you have ahead of time an idea of what to expect after your baby is born. If you aren't familiar with the hospital, ask your doctor what the procedures are for lying-in and, if possible, visit the hospital with your husband. Many hospitals today have arrangements for rooming-in (that is, keeping the baby with you); others have modified rooming-in plans, whereby you can have your baby with you when you wish, and return him to the nursery when you're tired. There are emotional advantages to the early closeness rooming-in makes possible, but there's no point in forcing such a relationship if you're too exhausted to care easily for the baby.

Find out what visiting hours are, how long your husband can stay with you and how many other visitors are allowed. (With full rooming-in, visitors are usually limited to the father and one or two other adults.) There's presently a trend toward shorter stays in the hospital, so it's probably just as well if you don't plan to see everyone you know. You'll have plenty to do in the little time you have. However, if you've been delivered by Caesarian, and have to stay in the hospital for about a week, you might appreciate more visits.

*A mother kisses five perfect
toes, and the toes respond with
a healthy grasping reflex.*

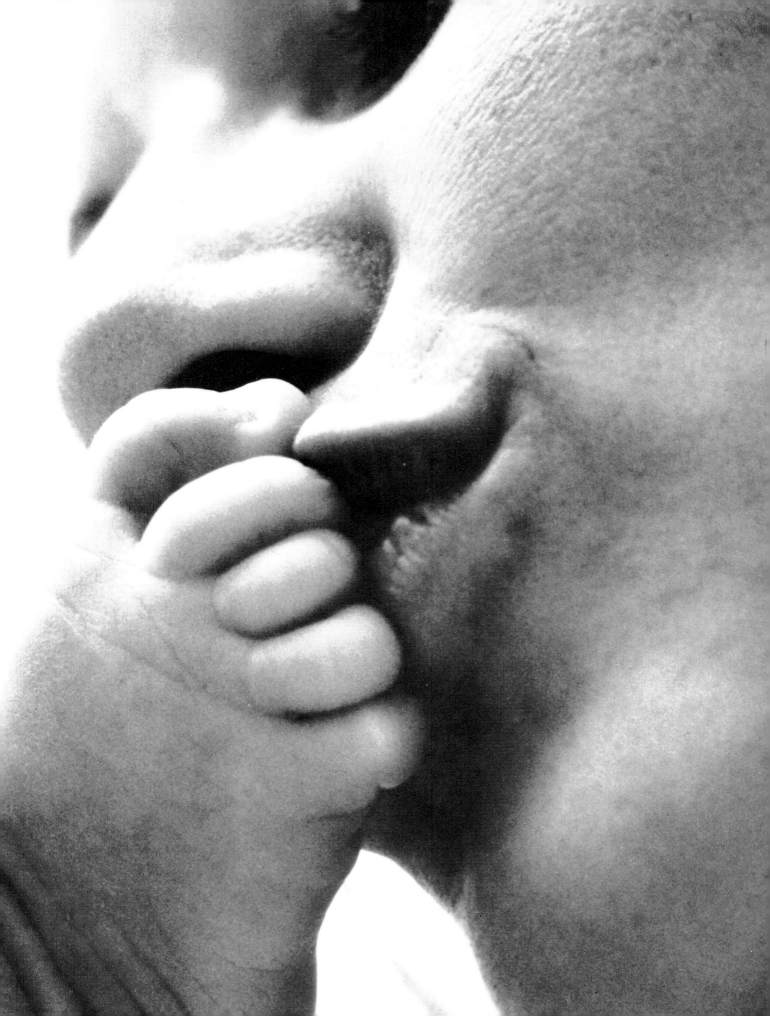

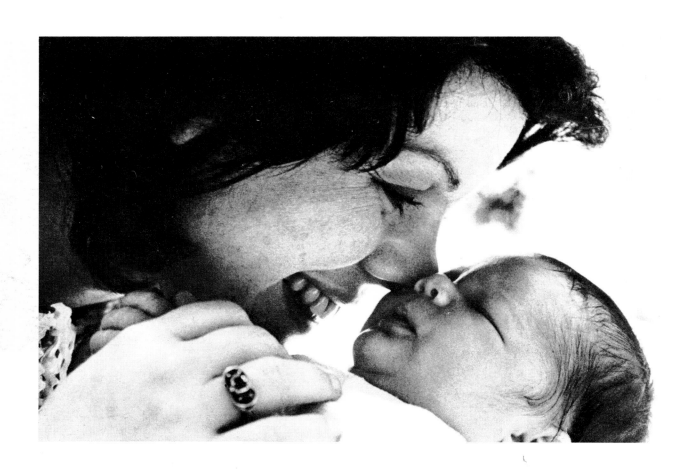

The average stay in the hospital for normal delivery is four days. If you'd like to leave sooner—for financial or other reasons—speak to your doctor. He may not object. Many women, however, often overestimate the strength they're going to have following birth, and appreciate and need the four days' rest.

Most hospitals bring the baby to the mother every four hours for feeding (including the 2:00 A.M. feeding if she wants and is strong

A baby sleeps with a small smile, enchanting her mother.

126

Lying-in floors are usually cheerful and busy.

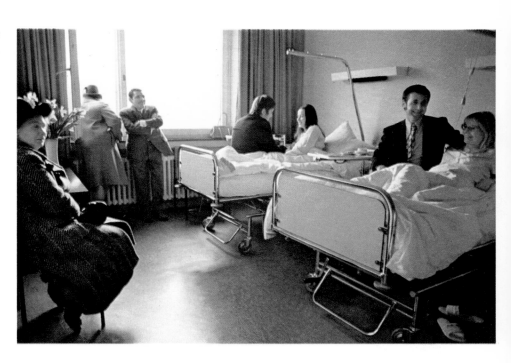

enough). The baby stays about an hour. The father can be there for at least some of the feedings.

Whatever arrangement your hospital has, it probably won't suit you perfectly. You'll have to put up with some necessary inconveniences. But you don't have to put up with *un*necessary inconveniences. If you're worried or upset about some aspect of the hospital routine, speak up. Hospitals do tend to be demoralizing. Women (and men) who hold down responsible jobs in the outside world may suddenly feel dependent and timid when they're in a hospital. A recurring problem is a mother seeing her baby crying in the nursery and feeling she can't do anything because it isn't feeding time. Don't stand there with tears in your eyes, feeling helpless. Speak to the

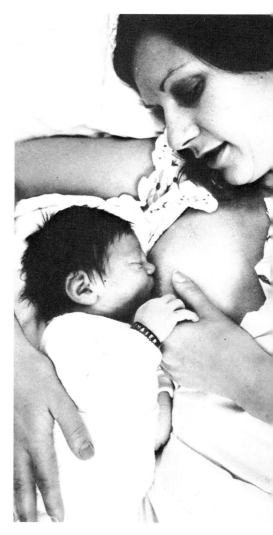

nurse in charge of the nursery. Perhaps the baby can be brought to
you early. Maybe he needs a diaper change. If you're reasonable, you
should be able to establish a good working relationship with most of
the nurses. If you're not satisfied, speak to your doctor, midwife or
pediatrician. If you're tired and shaky and not sure of your judg-
ment, ask your husband to speak for you and try to work out a solution.

The best approach is to ask the nurses questions. Most will respond warmly once they realize you respect their expertise and will
listen to their advice. And they can make your stay much easier. For
example, your baby may be fussy and worrying you no end just
because you're not burping her adequately. Every baby nurse has
good methods for getting up air.

The focus of most parents' anxiety about caring for a newborn is
on feeding. More and more mothers feel that breast feeding is preferable, because breast milk is the ideal food for babies, leading to few
problems with allergic reactions or indigestion; because the act of
nursing is emotionally rewarding for mother and child; because
breast feeding is in many ways more convenient and, finally, because
breast-fed babies are generally more content. Some mothers fear to
start the baby on the breast, because they imagine that they'll never
be able to get away from the baby for more than an hour or two. But
actually you should make a point of giving a breast-fed baby a bottle
now and then; otherwise, in an emergency (if you were to become ill,
for example), the baby might refuse the bottle. Many women feel
that, far from tying them down, breast feeding allows them more
freedom—no worries about bottles and warmers, mixing formula and
sterilizing equipment.

On the other hand, none of the arguments for breast feeding are
important if the process is making the mother and baby unhappy.
There are any number of reasons why it may not work out for a particular mother and child. If you can't or don't want to breast feed,

*When a newborn nurses, his
face expresses absolute concen-
tration.*

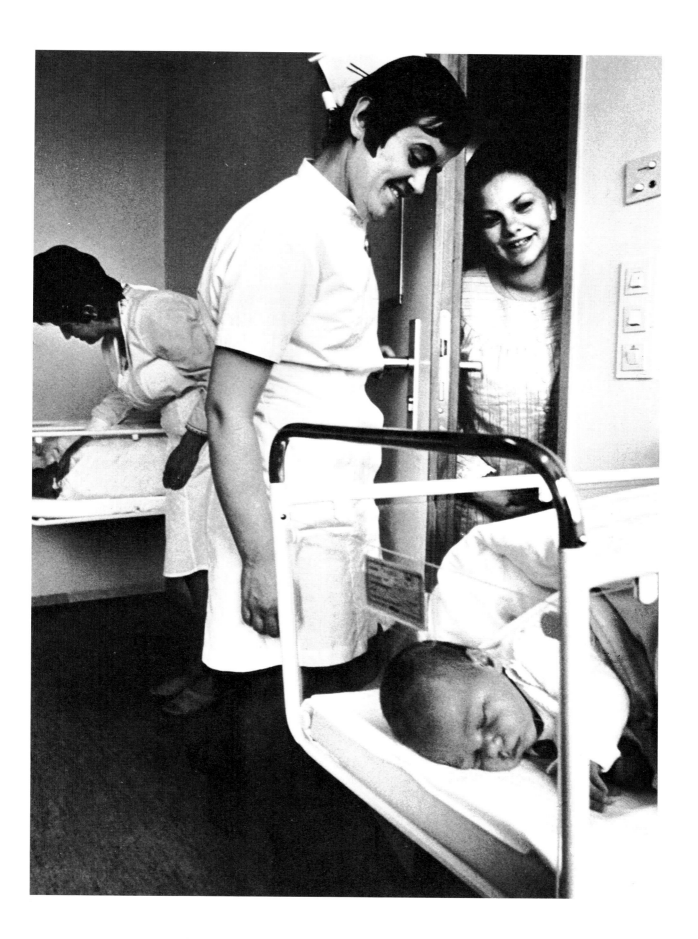

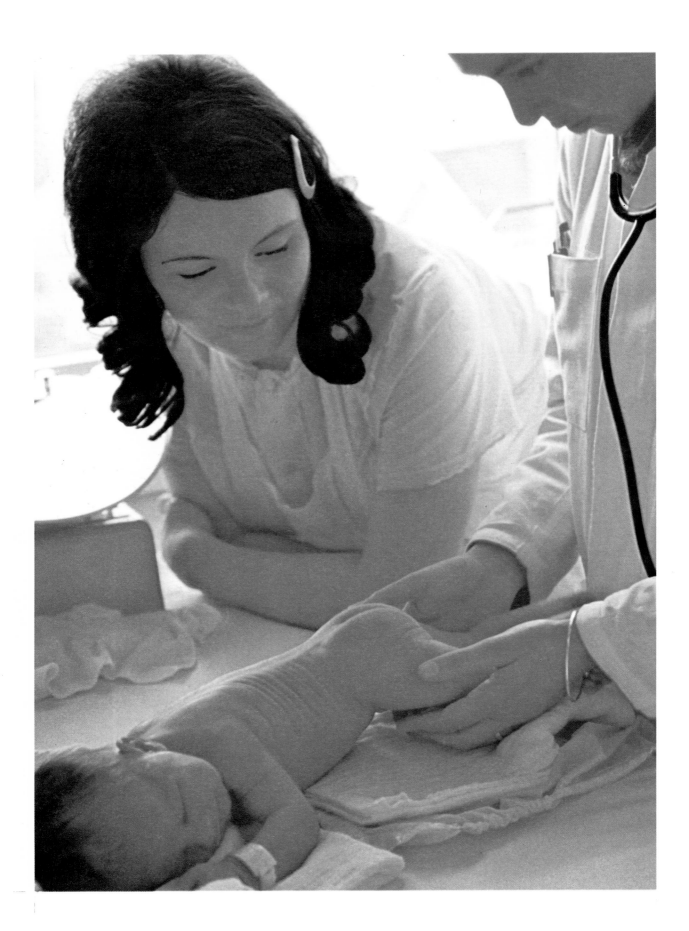

give the baby a bottle and tell well-meaning friends who make critical comments to come back another day.

If you do plan to breast feed, it's smart to read one of the many good books on the subject. Some women imagine they ought to know all about nursing by instinct, but it doesn't work that way. Learning and practice are needed.

There are two common mistakes that new mothers make that the nurses in the hospital will help you with. 1) A nursing baby doesn't suck on the breast's nipple, and a baby should never be allowed to do this. He can hurt you. Instead, he takes the whole areola into his mouth. By pressing the edges of the areola he expresses the milk. If you've ever milked a cow or seen one milked, you know you don't pinch the end of the teats. You massage further up, and the milk flows out in a stream. 2) The baby doesn't nurse with his lips pursed, as if he were sucking on a straw. A nurse should show you how to fit the breast to the natural shape of the baby's mouth. This is done by placing your thumb and index finger at the outer edge of the areola, above and below the breast. Press until the areola has a flatter shape, corresponding to the shape of the baby's mouth. Give the whole areola to the baby; he should latch right on.

For babies who won't feed, some nurses have a variety of other tricks, such as putting sugar water on the nipple. But the best trick of all is patience and calm. Don't worry if your baby takes a while to get started. You two will have plenty of time to learn together. Many parents imagine that the baby is ravenous after birth and eager to fill up on milk. Not at all. In fact, for the first few days your "milk" is really colostrum (a thin yellow liquid), which contains antibodies and is mildly cathartic. So there's no rush to become an expert breast feeder. Your baby will become expert when he's truly hungry.

Care of yourself after childbirth is primarily aimed at regaining strength and avoiding infection. You may have some pain where the episiotomy was stitched and "afterpains," which are contractions of

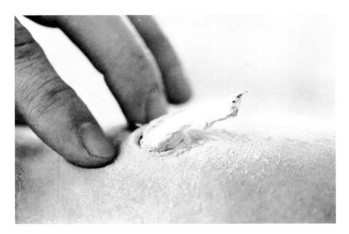

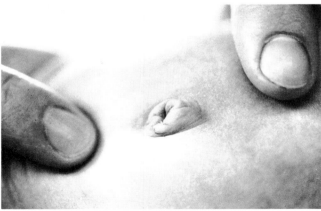

The dried-up end of the umbilical cord will fall off in about a week. When the wound is completely healed, the baby can have a real bath. Eventually the skin will pucker and probably turn inward.

the uterus as it shrinks back to its previous size. The hospital will give you some sort of analgesic, such as aspirin with codeine, to make you comfortable. Also a warm bath and heat lamp are soothing for the vaginal area. If these aren't suggested, ask for them. There is usually some bleeding for a period of a few days to a couple of weeks, which is why you should have sanitary pads on hand. Tampons are prohibited because of the chance that they might introduce an infection and irritate the episiotomy. You may also be given special moist

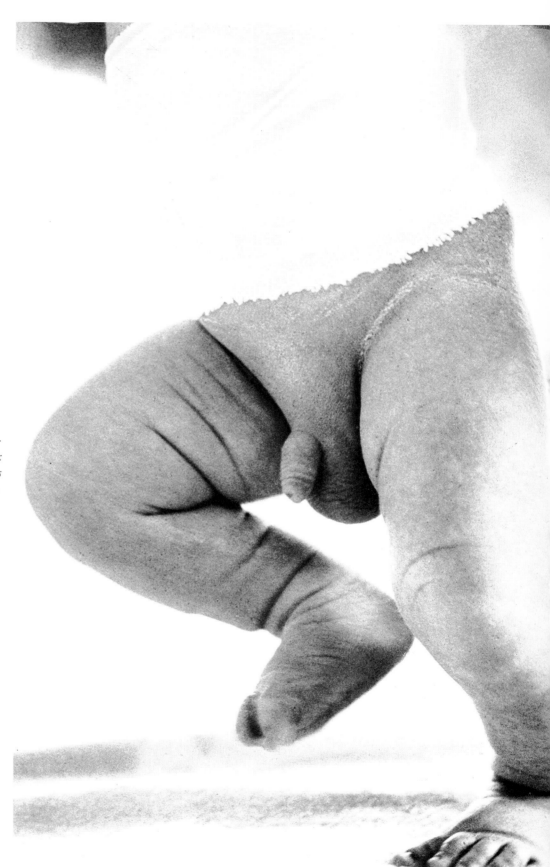

This baby is demon-strating the "walking" reflex that is normal among newborns but doesn't last.

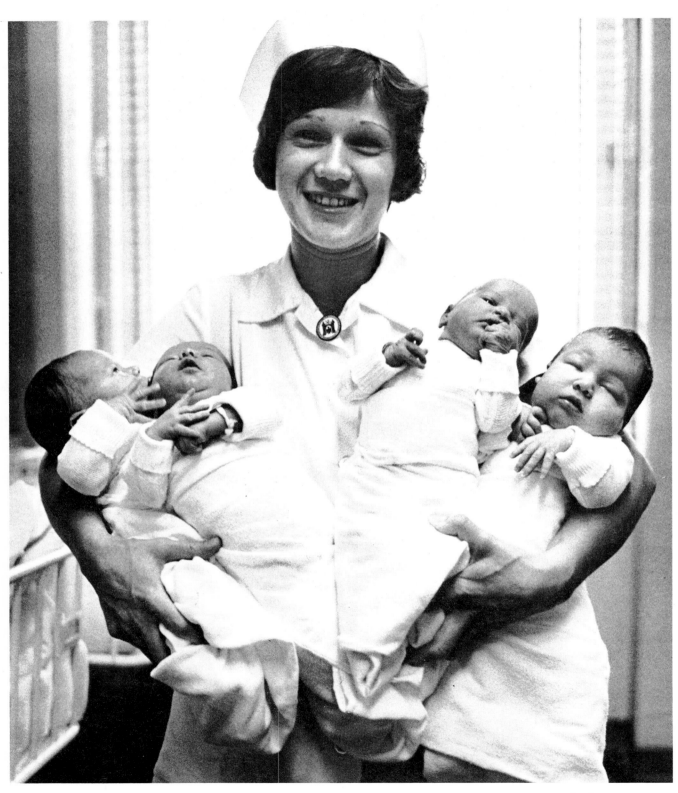

Maternity nurses have the happiest work in the hospital.

New parents make slow progress on their way home. The baby must be admired every few minutes.

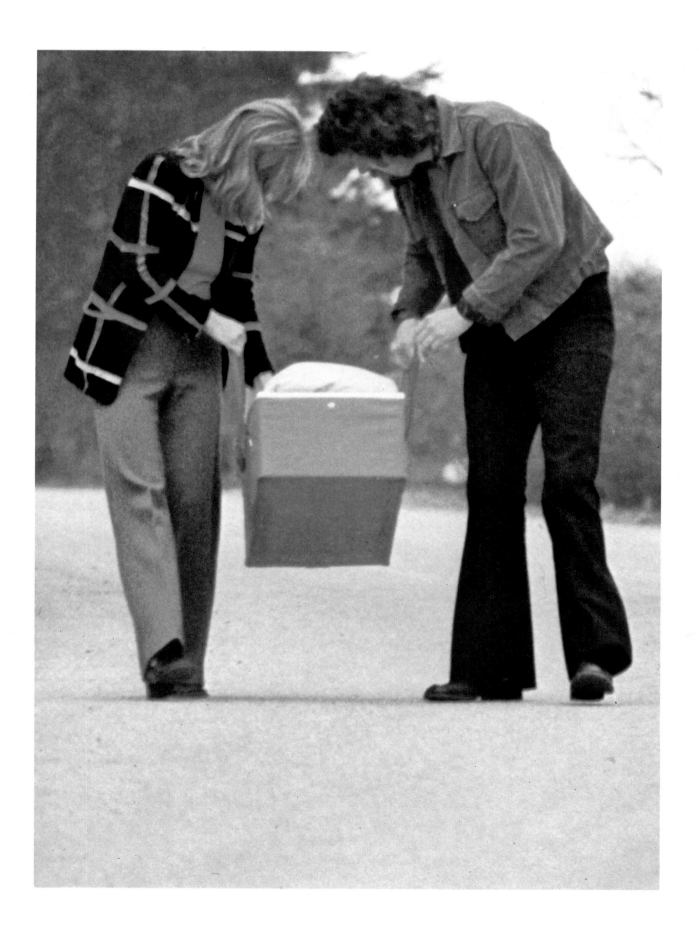

wiping tissues for cleaning yourself after using the toilet (always wipe away from the vagina, never from the anus forward toward the vagina). And the hospital may provide a small irrigating bottle, which you can fill with warm water. The water can be squeezed out in a stream for rinsing off while you're sitting on the toilet. It's handy for freshening up.

To regain tone in your vaginal muscles and the related muscles of the urethra and rectum, start doing Kegel (perineal-tightening) exercises as soon after delivery as possible, even before you're taken back to your room. If you've taken prepared-birth classes, you'll probably have been taught these; if not, ask your doctor or midwife or one of the nurses to explain them. Basically, they're just a flexing and release of the vaginal muscles: Tighten your vaginal muscles until the vagina is closed as much as possible. Hold the muscles tight for three or four seconds, then release. Then tighten again. Do this at least ten times, three times a day. These exercises are important for preventing problems that may arise later in life from loss of muscle tone. They also help right away to restore the tone of the vagina. Many women are extremely anxious that childbirth will stretch the vagina and they'll no longer be sexually desirable. This fear is usually much exaggerated. Cleopatra, Catherine the Great and Elizabeth Taylor all had babies. Nevertheless, it is true that giving birth affects the vagina, so the Kegel exercises are highly recommended. In fact, they're beneficial to any woman.

When you get home you can start leg-raising exercises to strengthen the abdomen. You should continue these until you're satisfied your stomach is firm.

Discuss with your doctor when you can resume sexual intercourse. Most doctors recommend waiting at least two weeks or until all bleeding has stopped. The idea is to avoid infection and allow proper healing of the episiotomy. You may be dismayed to find that you're not as eager to resume sexual activity as you imagined. This is probably partly because of worry over the new baby and possibly also because of temporary hormonal changes. In a couple of months you'll feel more like yourself.

The most common mood change after birth is a period of depression. This is traditionally said to coincide with the coming-in of milk, a couple of days or so after delivery. The mother suddenly starts crying or feeling very sad and irritable. Physiological factors probably cause some of the depression; other relevant factors probably include fatigue and anxiety. The depression can come right after birth or a week or two later—or not at all. If you do start feeling miserable, don't be alarmed. Protect yourself. Tell your husband to get rid of unwanted visitors. Don't push yourself into doing unnecessary chores. Treat yourself to some lazy distraction you enjoy, reading a mystery or watching a daytime movie on TV. You should be fine in a couple of days.

If the depression is severe and lasts for more than a week or two tell your doctor, and if he isn't responsive and helpful, find one who is. If you really feel bad and don't snap out of it, this is more than the standard "blues."

If you've been looking forward to the day you take your baby home, your happiness will touch many people near you. When parents leave a hospital with a new baby, passers-by look and smile. At this moment, people share sweet feelings. The baby is usually wrapped in a magnificent blanket fit for royalty, and the parents carry her as if she were crystal. They are taking their child to her home. The baby is beginning her life in a family. In the parents' faces there is pride, love and concern.

That day you will look at your baby and think, "There never was another baby like this." And you'll be right.

Prepared Childbirth

Today, more and more couples, especially those having their first child, are considering the various methods of "prepared childbirth." This interest reflects the concern in the United States at this time about health and physical fitness. Prospective parents want to minimize the amount of medication received by the mother and baby during labor and, in general, they're worried about any unnecessary intervention in the progress of labor and birth. Also, women are having fewer children and trying to develop the best possible relationship with these children. Mothers and fathers want to welcome their baby together and start caring for him as soon as possible. They want to get away from birth experiences that are so devastating (or are made to seem so) that the mother has to be knocked out and the father is sent away. As more and more parents experience joyful births, it is clear that traumatic labors should be considered the exception.

In the recent past the term "natural childbirth" has been used for various techniques of preparing women for the process of labor and birth. The term, which was coined in 1932 by Dr. Grantly Dick-Read of Great Britain, is actually a misnomer. A completely "natural" childbirth would be one the woman experienced without any form of medical intervention or previous planning. In "prepared" childbirth the mother and usually the father are educated and trained in techniques of coping with labor, and they are assisted by medical personnel.

Classes to prepare for childbirth are available in most regions of the United States. They are usually taught by a registered nurse or a woman who has been through a delivery using the techniques being taught or by a husband and wife team (in the Bradley method). Typically the courses consist of weekly sessions of one to two hours for four to eight weeks, usually in the last trimester of pregnancy. This time in pregnancy is chosen because as birth nears a couple is increasingly motivated to learn about childbirth and to practice the exercises.

The classes may be given at the instructor's home, at a doctor's office or at the hospital where you will deliver. Instructors usually are certified by one of the major maternity-centered organizations such as the American Society for Psychoprophylaxis in Obstetrics (ASPO), The International Childbirth Education Association (ICEA) or Maternity Center Association (MCA). An instructor will probably have received classroom instruction in the method, have observed numerous women in labor, acted as a monitrice (labor coach) and passed various written and oral exams in order to qualify for certification.

Fees for classes vary widely. There may be no charge if the classes are part of a prenatal, labor and delivery package. For small private classes, most organizations suggest the fee should be ten percent of the obstetrician's fee. In hospitals the fees are usually less, the classes somewhat larger.

The main goal of these classes is to discuss pregnancy, labor and delivery clearly and thoroughly, so that you will understand what is happening and what will happen to your body. A woman who has this information can greatly assist those caring for her by helping them to identify significant physical changes. Moreover, the woman who understands the process of birth has already conquered some of the fear and anxiety that can make childbirth far more difficult than it need be.

Most women ask particularly about the quality and intensity of labor contractions. A woman having her first child naturally wants to know what the experience of labor will be like, how painful it will be and whether she'll be able to stay in control of the process. Women having a second child can be assured that this one is probably going to be easier, and once labor starts most of these women say with relief that the contractions are milder than before. This is partly because the cervix has become more relaxed, but—probably more important—the woman goes into labor knowing that she can successfully give birth. She may still experience pain but she doesn't tense up so much.

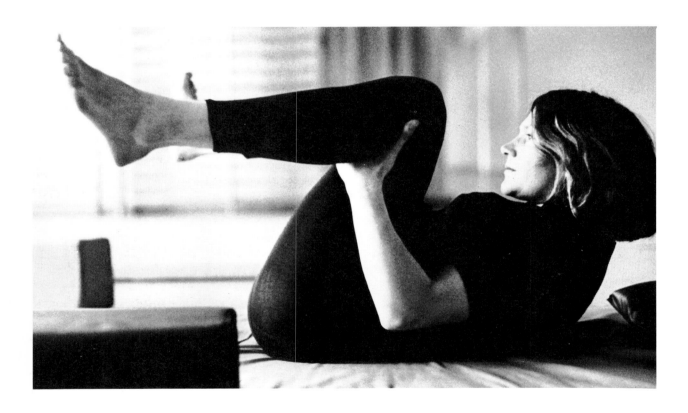

The psychological aspect of labor is extremely significant. Your attitude can be paramount in the perception of pain. When a toothache is torturing you, nothing is worse than clenching your teeth. This isn't to say that the pain of a toothache or labor is "in your mind" or "just psychological." But some ways of reacting to pain make it worse and others relieve it. Labor contractions are muscular tensings, like cramps, and anxiety tends to increase their intensity. Not understanding what's happening in labor, being treated unsympathetically, being frightened—all lead to tension and discomfort. Education and understanding tend to dispel the anxiety.

Modern women don't have much of a chance to learn about child-

This woman is practicing pushing by holding her breath and bearing down. The exercise strengthens the abdominal muscles.

birth in their daily lives. Birth takes place away from the comforts of home in the technological maze of a hospital. Given the success of contraceptive techniques, there are fewer pregnant women around to talk to and learn from. When a woman conceives her first child she may feel unique and alone. In her isolation from other pregnant women, she has little chance to discuss the worries that are universal to all pregnant women—fear of harm to oneself, fear the baby will be injured or ill, diffuse feelings of concern about becoming a parent. One of the advantages of attending classes in childbirth is the chance to get to know other pregnant women and women who have given birth before.

Many methods of relieving pain in childbirth have been tried throughout the millennia. The modern era of labor analgesia and anesthesia is sometimes dated from 1853, when Sir James Clark and Dr. John Snow gave Queen Victoria whiffs of chloroform during the birth of her child Leopold. But the pioneering doctor in pain relief was the most renowned obstetrician of the day, Sir James Young Simpson, who started using ether and chloroform in 1847.

The basic concepts of prepared birth were evolved by Dr. Dick-Read early in this century after he had attended a woman in labor who refused the chloroform he offered. Later, when he asked her why she didn't take it, her response was that the labor hadn't hurt. And then she asked, "It wasn't meant to, was it?" From this incident, he eventually formalized a theory, which he explained in his book *Natural Childbirth* (1932). Simply, he hypothesized that not understanding labor or knowing what to expect resulted in fear, and fear caused generalized body tension. This tension, he believed, hindered the natural physical process of birth and resulted in the experience of pain. He therefore established a series of lectures for pregnant women, to educate them, to help them to relax and give in to the activity of labor, to help them overcome the discomfort. He also taught certain exercises and breathing techniques to prepare the

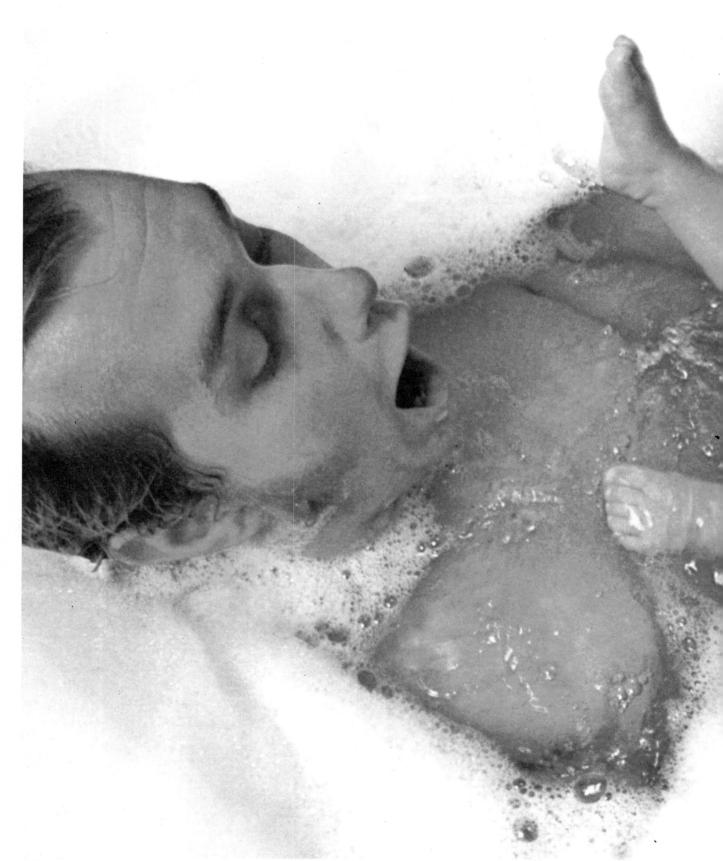

This father was present at the birth of his daughter, and they've been good friends ever since.

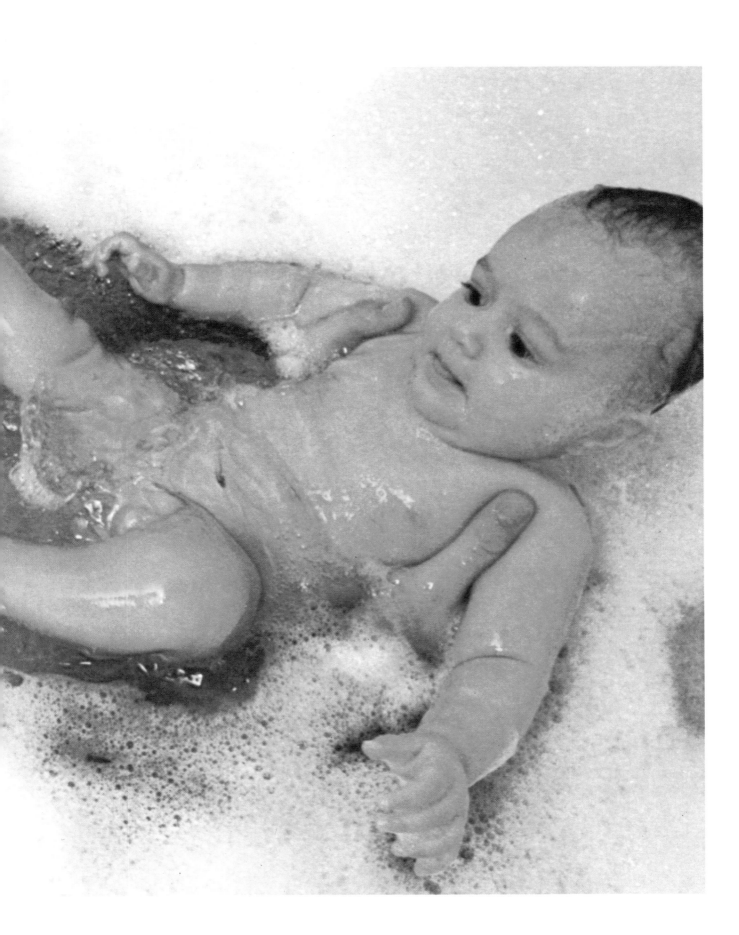

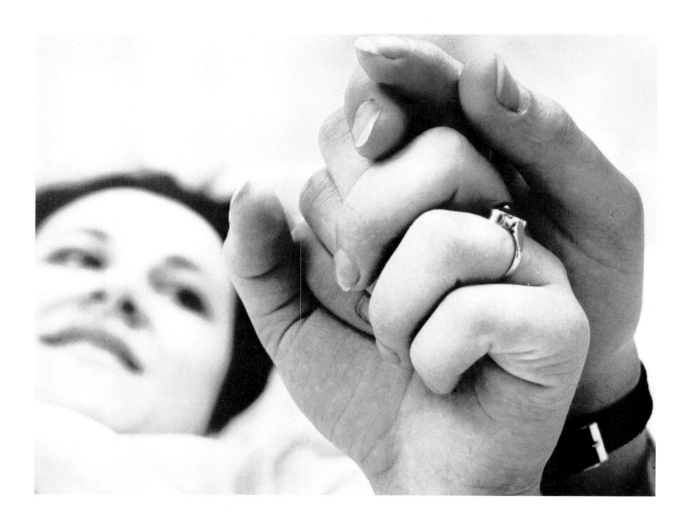

woman physically. With his approach, Dr. Dick-Read hoped not only to lessen pain but to restore women's dignity in childbirth.

The physical techniques involved slow abdominal breathing during the first stage of labor and deep muscular relaxation. Dr. Dick-Read also taught his patients how to assist their contractions during the second stage by holding their breath (to increase the intra-abdominal pressure) and pushing out the baby.

Today, most women study a somewhat different approach, the Lamaze method, which was first developed in the USSR, and is based on Pavlov's concepts of conditioning. During the 1930s in Russia, there was a shortage of doctors, and a program of breathing techniques was evolved to ease labor discomfort. In this program, the

The father's encouragement and comfort are invaluable in labor.

woman trained herself to respond to the stimulus of a contraction with a specific breathing response, rather than by tensing or saying "ow" or the like. The breathing response is learned by rigorous training and becomes automatic—contraction means breathe.

In the 1950s, Dr. Fernand Lamaze introduced the Russian methods in France. As the doctor for the metal workers' union in Paris, he had visited the USSR and observed the success with which women there were controlling their own labors. Combining the Russian techniques with a program of instruction adapted from Dick-Read's work, he began teaching women to prepare for childbirth. Marjorie Karmel brought the word about the benefits of a Lamaze birth to the United States with her book *Thank You, Dr. Lamaze* (1959), which is still popular today. It's a good first-hand account of giving birth by the Lamaze method. It also describes the problems she encountered when she attempted to find a doctor in New York who would be willing to allow her to use these techniques.

A very important aspect of Lamaze instruction is that the father is usually trained to participate as the wife's coach in childbirth. Because of his close concern for her and the baby, he is generally more effective than an outsider in responding to her and giving comfort and support. And her trust in him helps her to have confidence in his encouragement and guidance.

The mother and father who have prepared for childbirth should be backed up by a physician or midwife and hospital staff who are versed in the Lamaze method. The ideal is a well-coordinated team. The labor nurse should know how to help the husband support his wife and be able to explain what's happening when conditions vary from what the parents have learned in class. She should also understand that in the excitement of the moment the couple may briefly forget facts, procedures and techniques that they've studied for weeks. A gentle reminder—not exasperation—is what's called for.

If the nursing staff isn't familiar with the Lamaze approach, it may be advisable to have a labor coach, or monitrice, present. Some couples are afraid that a monitrice will usurp the role of the husband in guiding his wife, but this shouldn't happen. The monitrice should augment and help the husband. She can provide reassurance as new situations arise. Since no two labors are exactly alike, an experienced person on the scene can be very welcome. She provides continuity if there's a change of shifts during the labor, and she should be effective and tactful in explaining hospital procedures to the parents and in conveying the parents' concerns to the staff.

The doctor or midwife managing the birth also should feel responsible for helping the couple achieve the experience they hope for. This doesn't mean leaving the parents alone "to do their own thing." On the contrary, the doctor or midwife should be present and supportive and should give information willingly about the course of labor as it progresses. Managing a prepared birth is often more time-consuming than, say, speeding up the labor with Pitocin and then anesthetizing the woman when the pain becomes a problem. And this is why it's a good idea if you're interested in Lamaze to check with other patients of your obstetrician, to be sure that he or she is genuinely committed to this approach. There are, of course, some doctors who go along with it as long as it makes their lives easier, but who aren't willing to put in extra time or effort.

The Lamaze method is usually taught in six sessions of two hours each during the last trimester of pregnancy. If the father is not to be your coach in labor, you can choose another person, such as your mother or a friend. During the course you may have the chance to see a movie of a Lamaze delivery and to visit your hospital and meet some of the staff members. One of the most pleasant experiences for the class, if it can be arranged, is a visit from a couple who have recently delivered using the Lamaze technique. You can see that other people like yourself were able to use the method effectively and to enjoy the birth of the child together. These couples are also very sensitive to the questions of prospective parents and have the very

The father acts as a labor coach, guiding his wife in the correct breathing techniques for different phases of labor and keeping her company during the long hours.

146

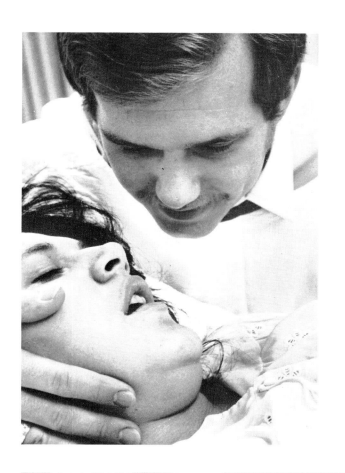
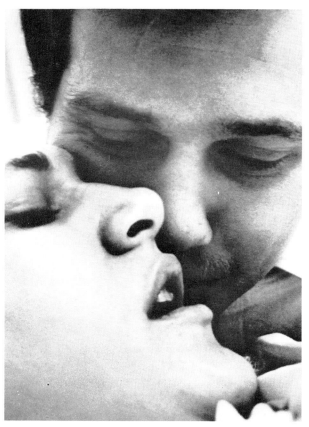
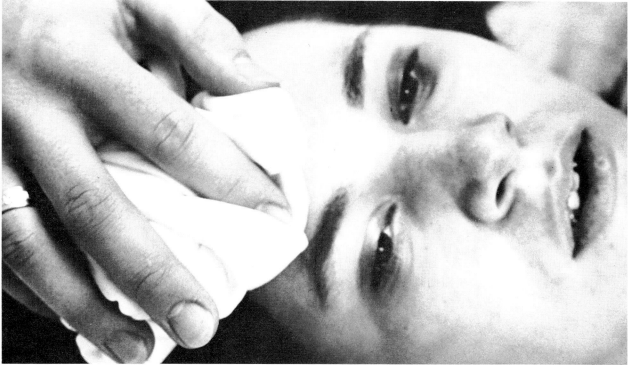

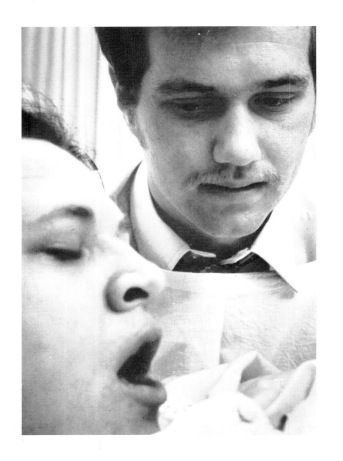
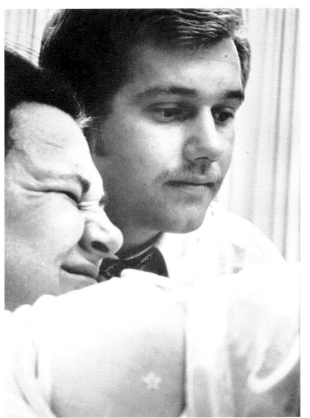
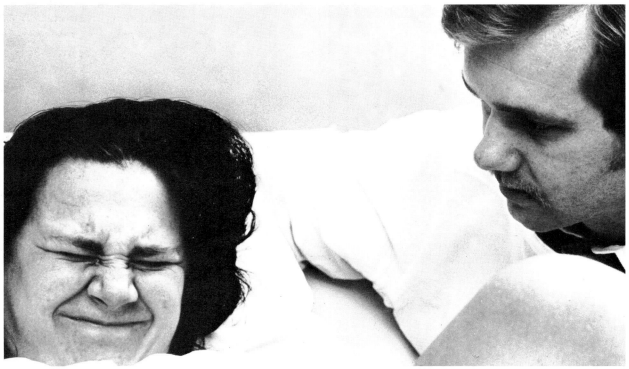

latest information about what it's like in the hospital.

Lamaze instruction covers four broad areas: the anatomy and physiology of pregnancy; normal labor and delivery; physical exercises; and specific breathing techniques. In the discussion of pregnancy, emphasis is placed on explaining the causes of what you may be experiencing, such as shortness of breath or Braxton-Hicks contractions. You should ask questions about any symptoms you have that you've wondered about. Probably other women in the group have had the same concerns. In discussing labor and birth, the course should cover not only what will happen physically, but what to expect in the hospital in the way of preps, enemas, tests, and who will be with you and what their responsibilities are. Ask questions until you feel confident that you understand how the hospital works.

In the classes you will be taught how to identify labor and how to assess its progress, so that you won't have to worry about not making it to the hospital in time. This is one of the most common worries and least common occurrences.

In your classes you should learn that you will have encouragement, support and comfort in labor. Your partner, the nurses, the doctors will all be trying to help you.

To prepare yourself physically you'll be taught exercises to strengthen your abdominal muscles (such as leg lifts) and to stretch the thigh muscles (such as sitting in the tailor position, which stretches the ligaments joining the bones of the pelvis). Relaxation exercises, technically referred to as neuromuscular-control exercises, are given to help you develop conscious control of specific muscle groups. These are extremely important exercises, because they promote awareness of tension in the body and deliberate relaxation. You will use the awareness and control during labor contractions to relax your entire body, especially your hands, arms and legs.

All the exercises should be practiced for a brief time every day in order to derive their complete benefit.

The basis of the Lamaze method is a series of breathing exercises,

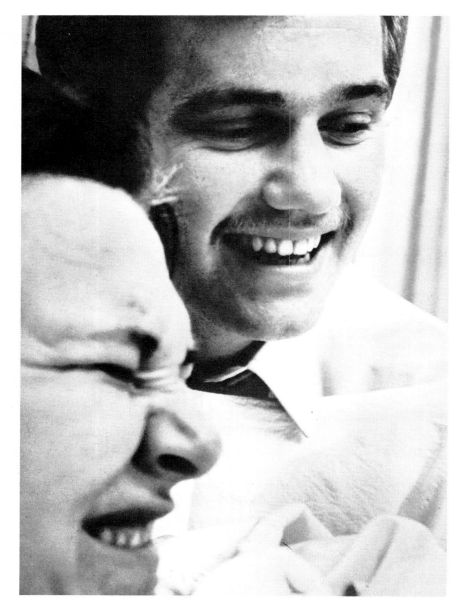

The baby's head has appeared. The mother is using all her strength. The father's excitement helps her to go on.

taught to the mother and her partner, or coach. The breathing techniques will help you ride over the discomfort of a contraction by focusing on the breathing response. You might doubt that mental activity affects how much discomfort you feel, but it does. For example, people who are greatly frightened, excited or happy don't seem to notice injuries that might ordinarily cause severe pain. Your mind and body can concentrate only on so much at one time. A football player in the Super Bowl who is concentrating on winning may not notice a broken bone. A woman in labor who is concentrating on her breathing and on relaxing is not so aware of discomfort. Moreover, the breathing exercises provide extra oxygen when the body needs it and therefore give you extra strength; in fact some women

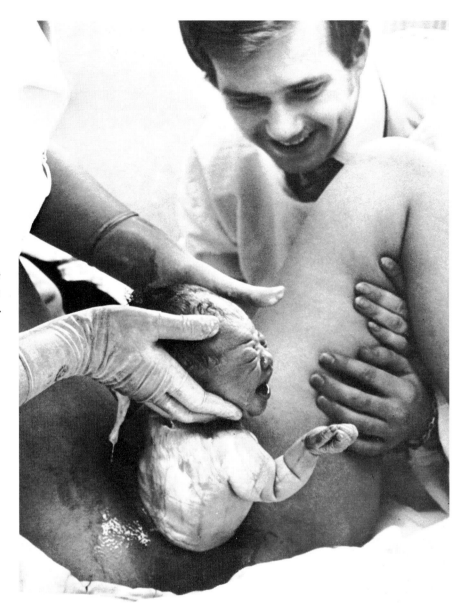

The baby is born. This is the moment of greatest exhilaration and joy.

notice that practicing the breathing exercises late in pregnancy rests and refreshes them, much as yoga breathing techniques do.

The exercises are progressive, from slow breathing for fairly easy labor to rapid breathing for late labor. They shouldn't be used until they're really needed, because they can become tiring or simply boring if done over a long period of time. The mother is usually reminded not to start her breathing techniques until she can no longer "walk-talk-or-joke" her way through a contraction.

Many couples have the mistaken idea that if you study a method of prepared childbirth, you will not or should not use any medications during labor or delivery. The proper role of breathing and relaxing

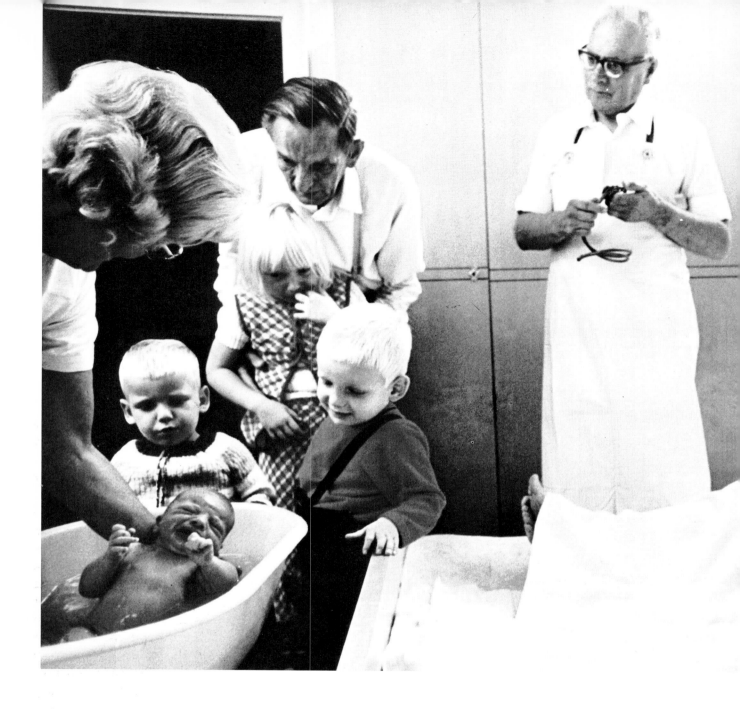

techniques is to give you more alternatives, not fewer, during labor. Don't hold out and refuse medicine if you really need it in order to cooperate in the labor and enjoy seeing your child born. Discuss with your partner and doctor ahead of time what your goals are and what kind of medication might be advisable under various circumstances. One of the great advantages of prepared childbirth is that thanks to the time you go without medicine, the baby and you should be in good shape to handle whatever pain relievers you might decide to use. If you do use medicine, it will be later and in smaller doses than would otherwise be needed. The goal is an alert baby and an alert mother, and moderate medication may be a help.

Demerol, the most frequently used pain reliever in labor, can work very well with the Lamaze method. One small dose may be suggested to help you in the final stages of cervical dilation, and then you will be completely conscious and at full strength during the time you're pushing out the baby.

If there is great discomfort, an epidural is an excellent solution, because you will be awake for the delivery. However, often forceps are needed, because the ability to push is diminished. It is usually best to try Demerol first, if you're having trouble getting through the contractions. This may be all the help you need. If you find it doesn't work well enough, you can still have an epidural.

Many women fear that if Pitocin is used to induce or stimulate labor, they won't be able to go through with Lamaze. It's true that this drug doesn't make labor any easier. Contractions induced by Pitocin are characteristically very regular, occurring every two to three minutes and lasting a uniform forty to fifty seconds. There isn't the slow onset of contractions and occasional slacking of contractions that occurs for brief intervals in a spontaneous labor. However, Pitocin does shorten the duration of labor, which can make the experience more tolerable. If you are well rested, though, you may go through induced labor without pain medication or with a minimal amount. At any rate, it's advisable to try the Lamaze techniques. For as long as they work, that's a benefit for the baby and you. And pain relief is available whenever you ask for it.

The most valued aspect of prepared childbirth is that the mother and father see and participate in the birth of their child. Their sense of accomplishment and excitement is usually beyond words. And fathers who have prepared have rightly earned their place in the labor and delivery rooms, for their encouragement and aid is extremely important to a successful delivery.

Many women consider taking classes and then don't act on the impulse because they decide they don't have the time. But the time you'll spend in classes is about the same amount of time you may spend in labor—not really long at all, but a very important time for your baby, a very important time for the whole family.

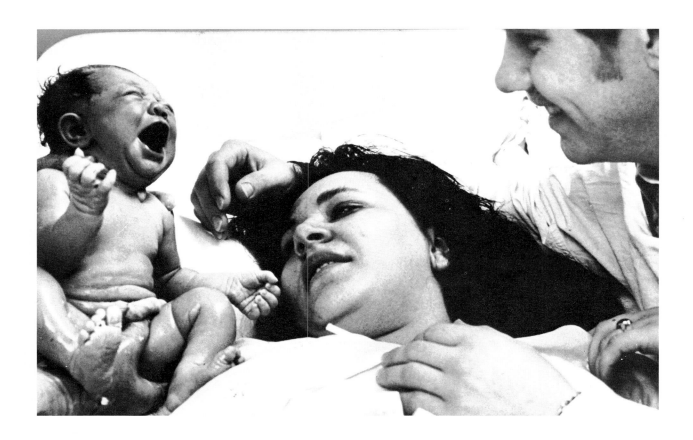

The following exercises are taught in Lamaze classes. The breathing techniques, particularly, can't be learned from a book. But a text is a good reminder for home practice.

NEURO-MUSCULAR CONTROL EXERCISES

Lie on the floor with a pillow behind your head and one under your knees for comfort. Legs should be slightly separated and arms should be resting on the floor by your sides. Eyes may be open or closed.

Your coach will check each arm for relaxation by securely grasping your hand, as if he were going to shake hands with you, and raising it from the floor with the elbow bent at a right angle. He should be able to feel the entire weight of your hand and arm, which should swing freely if swayed gently. If he lets go of your arm it should fall freely to the floor.

If he places his hands under one of your knees and gently lifts it, your leg should bend freely; it should be completely relaxed. Your knee should bounce gently as he moves it in his hands.

Now practice relaxation by contracting various combinations of muscles. To contract an arm, make a fist and raise the arm a few inches from the floor. When contracting your leg, flex the foot up at the ankle but do not raise it from the floor. Remember all limbs should be relaxed except those you are contracting. Also remember to relax the muscles in your face, and breathe.

EXERCISES: Contract right arm, relax
Contract right leg, relax
Contract left arm, relax
Contract left leg, relax
Contract right arm and right leg, relax
Contract left arm and left leg, relax
Contract both arms, relax
Contract both legs, relax
Contract right arm and left leg, relax
Contract left arm and right leg, relax

Your partner should give you directions using the specific commands above.

BODY-BUILDING EXERCISES

1. Sit on the floor with your legs crossed as long as possible to stretch your thighs and pelvic floor muscles. When you feel tired straighten your legs and shake them a bit and then resume the position. It is not necessary to keep your back straight; lean forward slightly so that the spinal column can relax.
2. Put the soles of your feet together and bend your knees, bringing your feet as close to your body as possible. Hold your ankles and bounce your knees up and down twenty times.
3. Lie flat on the floor with your legs extended and your arms resting at your sides. Begin by taking a *cleansing breath:* Inhale deeply through your nose and exhale through your mouth. Then point your

155

toe, raise your leg slowly as high as you comfortably can and inhale through your nose. Now, flex your foot, lower the leg slowly to the floor and blow the air out slowly through your mouth. Repeat with the other leg. Do this five times, alternating legs. Finish the sequence with another deep cleansing breath.

4. Lie on the floor, as in the above exercise. Take a cleansing breath. Raise leg, straight, with toe pointed as high as can be done comfortably and inhale. Flex foot and extend leg out to the side and toward the floor while exhaling. Point toe, bring foot back toward center and inhale. Flex foot, lower leg to floor and exhale through mouth. Repeat with other leg. Do exercise five times with each leg, alternating legs. Finish with a deep cleansing breath.

5. To strengthen abdominal muscles and relieve low backache, lie on floor with arms resting at sides, and bend legs at knees while keeping feet flat on the floor. Start by pushing the curve in your lower back to the floor and contracting your abdominal muscles, hold for a moment, then release. This will result in a slight rocking movement of the entire pelvic girdle. The coordinated breathing involves starting the exercise with an inhalation, then contract toward the floor while exhaling, release and inhale. Repeat five times.

6. To strengthen and gain control of the muscles of the pelvic floor, sit on a chair and contract the muscles around your urethra, vagina and anus; you will lift slightly off the chair. Hold for three or four seconds, then release. Repeat at least ten times each day. This exercise done daily after the baby is born will promote healing of your episiotomy, and if continued will maintain the tone of your entire pelvic floor.

NOTE: It is quite all right to do any other exercises that you are accustomed to doing, except sitting-up exercises. "Sit-ups" pull your abdominal muscles in the wrong sequence during pregnancy and should not be done from the time you have begun to "show" until after delivery.

LAMAZE BREATHING TECHNIQUES

Practice all the breathing exercises sitting slightly forward in a comfortable chair. When you are in labor you may walk around, sit in a chair or rest in bed on your side or with head and back supported by pillows.

Never practice lying in bed and never lie flat on your back in labor. This position will prevent proper expansion of your lungs, making it difficult to execute the techniques properly. Lying flat on your back also prevents proper flow of blood to the uterus and lower extremities.

TECHNIQUE 1: Take a cleansing breath, inhaling deeply through the nose and exhaling through the mouth. Focus eyes on a point directly in front of you. Slowly breathe in through the nose and exhale through the mouth, taking six to eight slow breaths in one minute. Coordinate with the breathing a slow massage of your abdomen, called effleurage—that is, the fingers rhythmically massaging the abdomen up as you inhale and down as you exhale. Finish the sequence with another cleansing breath.

Each breathing technique should be practiced at least three times each day. Simulate a contraction by having your partner time you for sixty-second intervals. He should say, "Contraction begins," then call out every ten seconds, "10, 20, 30, 40, 50, contraction ends." This way you will learn that the response to a contraction is to breathe.

Do not start using this technique in labor until you can no longer find any other way of distracting your attention. The movements should be very slow and relaxing.

TECHNIQUE 2: Take a cleansing breath, focusing your eyes on a point directly in front of you. Breathe entirely through your mouth or your nose, taking short breaths high in the chest and audibly expelling the exhalation. The inhalation should be soft and the exhalation forceful. You will be taking 80 to 100 short breaths per minute. Continue doing a slow effleurage of the abdomen while you breathe. Practice for sixty seconds and end the sequence with a cleansing breath.

Practice this exercise three times for sixty seconds each, taking short, even breaths. Then practice a change of pace, starting at a slow rate (60 per minute) and building to a fast rate (120 per minute) at about thirty seconds, and then decreasing the speed again. Always end with a cleansing breath.

During labor you will use this technique by starting at a slow rate when the contraction begins. As the contraction increases in intensity you will breath more rapidly and as it wanes you will again go back to a slow rate.

This technique is to be used only when the previous technique no longer helps you control your contractions. If you are examined by your doctor, who finds that you are not yet four centimeters, try and go back to the first slow breathing technique. Just finding out where you are in labor should help you relax a great deal and allow you the ability to concentrate better.

TECHNIQUE 3: Take a cleansing breath, focusing your eyes on a point directly in front of you. Take six short breaths high in the chest as in the previous exercise, then one strong, deep blow out. Repeat this pattern for sixty-second practice contractions. End with a cleansing breath. Do not do the effleurage with this exercise, but rest your hands comfortably on your lower abdomen. Practice this exercise three times each day.

Like the previous techniques, this exercise is to be used in labor only when absolutely necessary. Save it for strong contractions when you are at least seven centimeters dilated.

TECHNIQUE 4: To practice pushing for second stage of labor, lie on floor or bed with several pillows supporting your back. When contraction begins, take a deep cleansing breath. Take a second deep breath and hold it. Bring your chin toward your chest. Draw up your knees and hold them with your hands. Your elbows should be extended out and lifted high in the air at shoulder level. Bear down using the strength of your abdominal muscles while relaxing the muscles of the pelvic floor. When you cannot hold your breath any longer, remain in the same position, straighten your neck, exhale quickly and inhale again. Hold the breath and bring your chin forward again toward your chest. Repeat throughout the contraction. End the contraction with a cleansing breath. Your partner may assist by holding your feet up and pressing them toward your chest.

Remember that during the second stage of labor you should push only when you have a contraction. Do not be afraid to get into the pushing position and practice this exercise several times a day. During one practice contraction each day you may actually practice pushing with your full strength.

A Woman Gives

"I didn't want to let go of the child. I simply lay there, and my baby's forehead touched my throat. My baby was a girl—Julia."

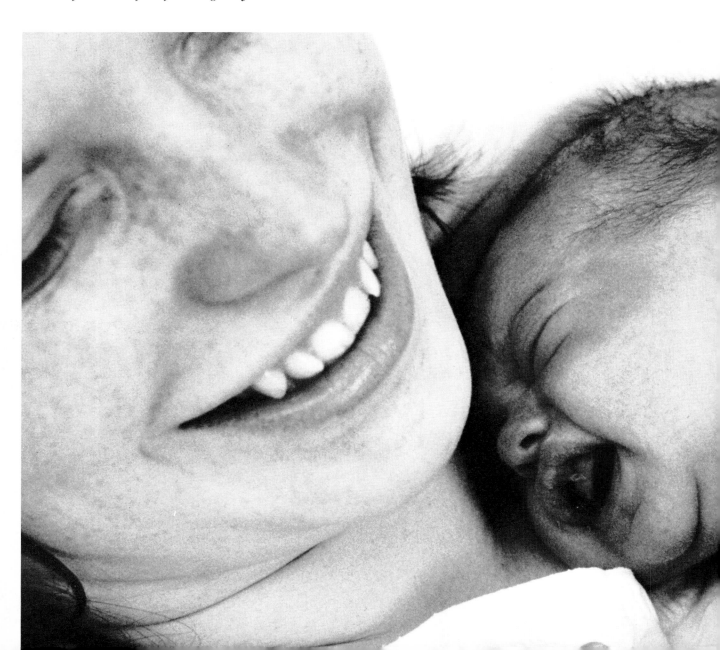

Birth Alone

"Before it was time to bear down and push, I was in agony. Screaming eased the pain. When I couldn't stand it any more, I was told to push. Push and pant. I felt no more pain. I was working with my whole body."

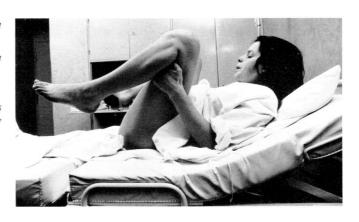

"During the pushing I had complete self-control. I breathed in, held my breath, pushed down. It was automatic. I felt the child passing out of my body."

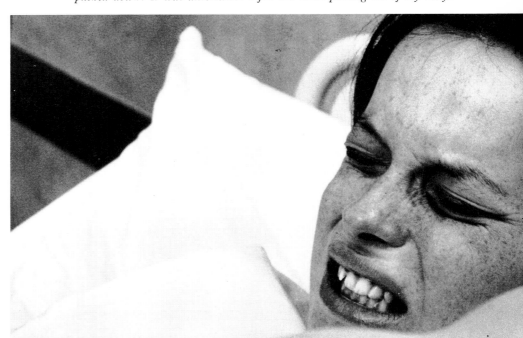

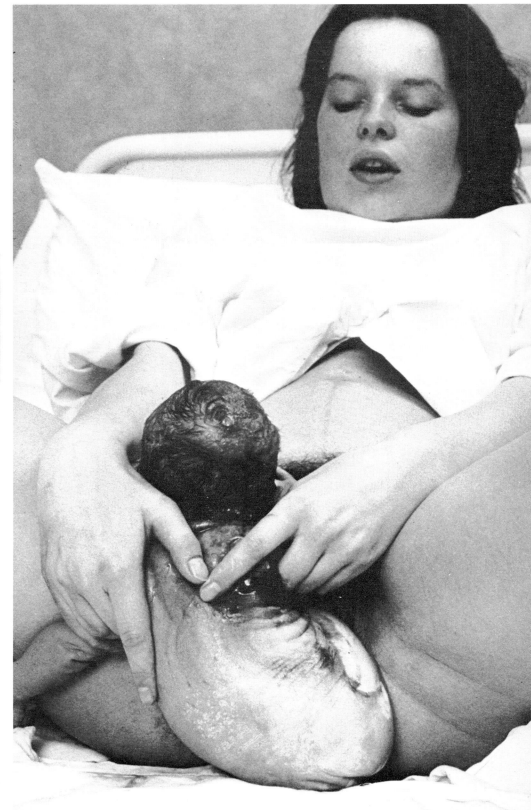

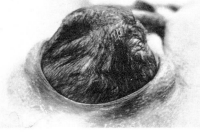

The child is almost born. The head has crowned. The rest will happen quickly.

" 'Now grab hold of it,' some-
one shouted. People pulled me
up and put pillows behind me.
I reached down. That animal
smell! I didn't really do any-
thing. I lifted something out,
that was all."

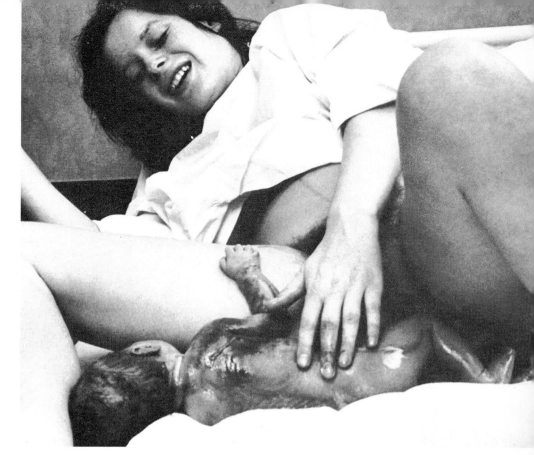

"When the baby lay between my legs, I wanted to leave it attached to the umbilical cord for a while and just look at it. I felt its warmth on my thighs. But the hospital people were making a commotion. I wouldn't have been in such a hurry if I'd been alone."

"They gave me gloves and a clamp and scissors. 'Where should I cut?' I asked. 'Any-where,' said a doctor. Even after the cord was cut, I still felt attached to my baby. I had no more pain. The afterbirth slipped out with a pang. There was a brief twinge when a small tear was stitched. Then they took the child away to examine and bathe her."

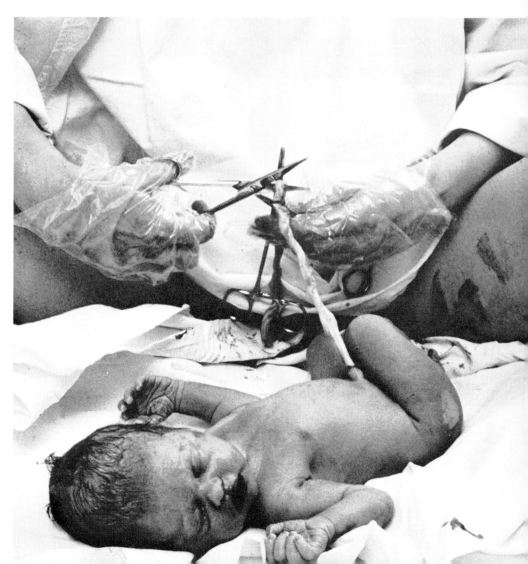

This woman gave birth to her daughter without a doctor's help. The birth was normal, as most births are. Nature delivered the baby safely. There was pain, laughter and love.

The woman had wanted to have her baby at home, but agreed to go to a hospital if she could deliver her baby herself. She wanted no one between her and her child. She listened to the advice of midwives, doctors and nurses, but she delivered her daughter with her own hands.

Not many women would be comfortable with this kind of experience. But it reminds us that a woman giving birth is not an invalid or patient, but a healthy person taking part in nature's creative process.

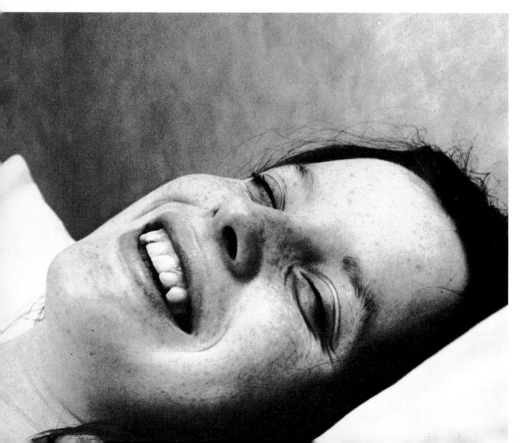

I was deliriously happy. I had to laugh. I just laughed and laughed.

Bibliography

Pregnancy and birth

BING, ELISABETH. *Six Practical Lessons for an Easier Childbirth*. New York: Bantam, 1969.

————. *Moving Through Pregnancy*. Indianapolis: Bobbs-Merrill, 1975.

BRADLEY, ROBERT. *Husband-Coached Childbirth*. New York: Harper & Row, 1965.

CHABON, IRWIN. *Awake and Aware*. New York: Delacorte Press, 1966.

DICK-READ, GRANTLY. *Childbirth Without Fear*. New York: Harper & Row, 1970.

EWY, DONNA AND ROGER. *Preparation for Childbirth*. Boulder, Colo.: Pruett Publishing Co., 1970.

FLANAGAN, GERALDINE. *The First Nine Months of Life*. New York: Simon & Schuster, 1962.

KARMEL, MARJORIE. *Thank You, Dr. Lamaze*. Philadelphia: J. B. Lippincott, 1959.

LAMAZE, FERNAND. *Painless Childbirth*. New York: Pocket Books, 1972.

Breast feeding

EIGER, MARVIN AND OLDS, SALLY. *The Complete Book of Breastfeeding*. New York: Workman, 1972.

LA LECHE LEAGUE. *The Womanly Art of Breastfeeding*. Franklin Park, Ill.: La Leche League International, 1963.

PRYOR, KAREN. *Nursing Your Baby*. New York: Harper & Row, 1973.

Childcare and development

BRAZELTON, T. BERRY. *Infants and Mothers*. New York: Delacorte, 1969.

FRIEBERG, SELMA. *The Magic Years.* New York: Scribner's, 1959.

KLAUS, MARSHALL H., AND KENNELL, JOHN H. *Maternal-Infant Bonding.* St. Louis: Mosby, 1976.

LEVINE, M. I., AND SELIGMANN, J. H. *The Parents' Encyclopedia.* New York: Crowell, 1973.

SALK, LEE. *What Every Child Would Like His Parents To Know.* New York: McKay, 1972.

SPOCK, BENJAMIN. *Baby and Child Care.* New York: Pocket Books, 1970.

Midwifery

ARMS, SUZANNE. *Immaculate Deception.* Boston: Houghton Mifflin, 1975.

HAIRE, DORIS. "The Cultural Warping of Childbirth." Seattle, Wash.: International Childbirth Education Association *News,* 1972.

Index